THE MALE

THE MALE
FROM INFANCY TO OLD AGE

Sherman J. Silber, M.D.

Illustrations by Scott Barrows

CHARLES SCRIBNER'S SONS · NEW YORK

2/1982
agni l

Copyright © 1981 Sherman J. Silber, M.D.

Library of Congress Cataloging in Publication Data

Silber, Sherman J.
    The male: from infancy to old age.
    Includes index.
    1. Andrology.   2. Generative organs, Male—
Diseases.   I. Title.
RC875.S57   612.6'9   81–40696
ISBN 0–684–17307–7   AACR2

3 5 7 9 11 13 15 17 19   F/C   20 18 16 14 12 10 8 6 4

Printed in the United States of America

Contents

Introduction

Over many years an attitude has developed that the female, with her menstrual periods, hormonal variations, and eventual menopause, is an incredibly complex creature, and that the male, in comparison, has a very simple sexual apparatus that functions tirelessly, without much complexity or any problem of serious breakdown. Mothers take a great deal of time to explain the facts of life to their daughters before the onset of menstruation, frequently emphasizing the terrible burden it imposes upon them. The complexity of their entire reproductive system is emphasized in television programs, in magazines that can be purchased in the grocery market, and even by the properly accepted ritual that women simply must submit at least yearly to a gynecological examination. With all this emphasis on female problems, the complexity of the male apparatus has not been sufficiently recognized. This has led to terrible frustrations for male patients who develop relatively common problems and are aghast to find out that perhaps their systems are not quite so simple after all.

For example, prostatitis in men between the ages of twenty and forty is almost as common an affliction as the cold. I hardly appreciated the emotional impact of this common infection until

I awoke one morning with an intense feeling of having to urinate, which was not relieved despite urination every fifteen minutes during the day. The penis had a swollen feeling to it, but looking at it revealed nothing unusual. I had to stand at the urinal for protracted periods before I could urinate at all, and then the emergence of a small amount gave me only temporary relief. Within fifteen minutes I had to urinate again. The thought of having sex seemed out of the question, and when I finally checked my own urinalysis and saw many red blood cells, I knew that I was finally about to undergo the ordeal that urologists such as myself consider routine for our patients.

As I lay there in the position that woman must endure at the time of their ritual gynecological examination, waiting for the anesthesia to take effect so that my colleague could place the cystoscope (which suddenly appeared to be incredibly long) through my penis into the bladder, I realized the great need for a book that would explain to the general public the complexity of the male reproductive system and its frequent disorders.

I recently saw a patient sitting in the corner of my examining room with the most guilty, depressed look I have even seen. I had been treating him during the past year for recurring prostatitis. Due to marital problems he was not having very much sex. I tried to ask him cheerfully how he was doing. He just looked sullenly at the floor and quietly whispered, "I've got it." The nature of his problem didn't completely hit me, because I see so many men who "have it," until he went on. "I knew I shouldn't have done it. It was just a stupid thing. I was sort of drunk and feeling sorry for myself." I asked him what it was that happened. He told me that he had not been able to have sexual relations with his wife for the past year and finally had had relations several nights before with a different woman. He then repeated, "I knew I shouldn't have done it, and now I've got it."

I examined his penis and saw that there was a very scanty discharge. He had minimal burning discomfort upon urination. His testicles and scrotum felt completely normal. I asked him to bend over and performed a rectal exam, palpating the prostate gland very carefully. The prostate was somewhat boggy and tender, no different from what I had found in this patient in the past. There was no evidence of venereal disease. His symptoms were actually caused by the fact that he had finally had intercourse after almost a year of abstinence. The woman with whom he had had intercourse was carefully checked and her cultures were also negative. Thus, the patient's problem was not that he had gone out and had intercourse and contracted venereal disease, as he had feared, but rather that he hadn't had intercourse frequently enough.

Production of sperm and testicular fluid is a complicated process, and the transport of this fluid up into the ejaculate via the secretions of the prostate and seminal vesicles is very complex. Any interference with the regularity of intercourse can have profound effects on this fluid and sperm transport. Also, the mere process of erection is so complicated that there still is a great deal of confusion among physiologists about exactly how the penis works. Psychological stresses can put it altogether out of commission temporarily. Distinguishing these psychological stresses from true physical causes of impotence is a critically important task. For the patient who performs poorly on a bad night, or who is under extreme duress from other causes and finds out that in addition he can no longer make love, the world can appear to be coming to an end. An accurate understanding of how the penis works, and what can be done to help this all-too-common situation, will go a long way toward solving the problem.

As one grows older, the frequency of sex and the intensity of sexual desire become subjects of great confusion. The fear of impotence or poor sexual performance afflicts every man at one time or another and becomes increasingly awesome for men over the age of fifty. Men and their partners are extremely resentful of the unconcerned and uninformed physician who just tells them not to worry about it.

Even if a man has been able to survive these perils of the penis through middle age, as he reaches his later years another problem inexorably emerges. His urinary stream begins to slow down and he has a difficult time emptying his bladder because of enlargement of the prostate. Then he has to worry about prostatectomy, incontinence of urine, dry ejaculation, and again impotence. Just the thought of having an operation performed through a telescope placed up through the penis, and having a catheter coming out through the penis for several days postoperatively until the bleeding has completely subsided, can be terrifying. Indeed, he has reason to be afraid, since cancer of the prostate is the third leading cause of death from cancer among men and is present in over 10 percent of men who undergo routine prostatectomy for a presumably benign disease. Cancer of the prostate is present in 80 percent of all men over the age of eighty.

The male genitalia are the subject of so much more confusion and pride than other parts of the body that even the most minor ailments can provoke an enormous array of terrifying fantasies. How does a mother deal with her ten-year-old son who is still bed-wetting? How does a new father decide whether or not his son should be circumcised? What about his three-year-old boy who is complaining that his erections hurt? Why does grandpa have to get up six times a night to urinate? Who does the twenty-year-old boy talk to when he has a drip from his penis? Who does his girlfriend talk to? What is puberty all about? Is your child a homosexual?

This book will serve as a guide for both men and women, to explain just how the male genitalia work, what can go wrong, and what can be done about it.

PART ONE
How the Male Organs Work

1

The Mechanics of Erection and Orgasm

The Structure of the Penis

The penis is basically composed of three parallel cylinders, all enclosed in an outer sheath of very stretchable, elastic skin. The two major cylinders (called the corpora cavernosa) that form the bulk of the erection lie side by side, and they extend all the way down to the bone that we sit on. An erect penis is thus supported by a firm foundation. Without this substructure to support the erection, the penis would wobble around and buckle during the in and out motions of intercourse. A third cylinder (the corpus spongiosum) surrounds the urethra, the channel through which both the urine and the semen squirt out.

During erection all three of these cylinders are engorged with so much blood that they become distended and rigid. Although the corpus spongiosum does not provide much support for the shaft of the penis, it is critical for supporting the tip of the penis during erection. The tip of the penis is where most of the sensory nerve endings for sexual arousal are located. Although stimulation of the shaft of the penis is helpful in sexual arousal, the greatest erotic sensitivity comes from the tip. Furthermore, the tip of the penis is very important in providing painless and streamlined penetration of the vagina.

The corpus spongiosum extends from the tip of the penis to the bulb, located just inside the base of the penis, between the two corpora cavernosa. This is where men feel the sensation of orgastic ejaculation. Two powerful muscles, the bulbocavernosus muscle and the ischiocavernosus muscle, surround this area. It is the contraction of these muscles around the corpus spongiosum and the bulb that provides the sensation of orgasm and squirts the semen out.

The inner structure of the corpora cavernosa (the cylinders of erection) consists of millions of minute, spongelike caverns supplied with blood by tiny vessels that pierce the dense, tough outer envelope surrounding the corpora. This internal skeleton fills with blood during arousal and creates a rigid, distended shaft. When the penis is flaccid, i.e., when there is no erection, the blood

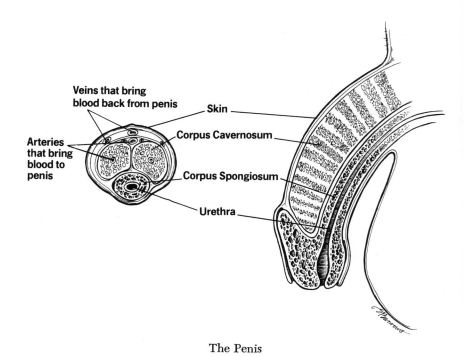

Veins that bring blood back from penis

Skin

Arteries that bring blood to penis

Corpus Cavernosum

Corpus Spongiosum

Urethra

The Penis

flow through it is minimal because millions of tiny sphincters are closed, preventing blood from entering the corpora. However, during sexual arousal, the little blood vessels open to allow huge amounts of blood to pour into the cylinders, providing a firm shaft for vaginal penetration. The system for controlling blood flow into and out of the penis, with an intricately timed interplay of opening and closing valves, is very complex and functions entirely without conscious thought.

Erection and Ejaculation

In order for this complicated experience of erection and ejaculation to occur, a system of nerve pathways is necessary to orchestrate the whole event. Erection is a reflex phenomenon over which the male has no direct voluntary control. He cannot will or demand an erection. There are two ways in which this automatic reflex can be stimulated. One is psychologically, through thought processes about sex, and the other is reflexly, through manipulation of the penis. A man cannot get an erection simply because he wants to have one.

There are three sets of nerves that supply the penis and control this phenomenon. One, the pudendal nerve, carries sensations from the penis to the spinal cord. From there sensations can either travel directly through motor nerves to the penis, resulting in a reflex erection, or go up to the brain, resulting in mental sexual arousal, which can in turn send motor impulses back down the spinal cord to the penis. Without pudendal sensory nerves, erections could not be caused by direct stimulation of the penis, but could be caused by mental arousal. The other two sets of nerves, the parasympathetic and sympathetic nerves, are motor nerves that control erection and ejaculation, respectively.

When the state of arousal becomes so intense that orgasm is inevitable, a message from the brain travels down the spinal cord to the sympathetic nerves, which pour out impulses that stimulate the muscles around the base of the penis to contract rhythmically, squirt out the semen, and provide the pleasurable sensation of orgasm.

Actually, what we commonly think of as orgasm comes in two distinct phases, emission and ejaculation. During sexual arousal and foreplay, sperm is quietly pumped from the scrotum through the vas deferens to the region near the ejaculatory duct (see below). The longer the period of foreplay and sexual activity, the greater the amount of sperm that is conducted slowly and quietly into this region. But there is no awareness of anything until the time of emission. Emission is that moment of "ejaculatory inevitability" when the seminal vesicles, located just behind the prostate gland, get ready to contract, and the sperm is squirted through the ejaculatory duct into the base of the penis. The seminal vesicles (which deliver most of the fluid but none of the sperm) contract and wash sperm through the ejaculatory duct into the bulb. Shortly thereafter ejaculation occurs.

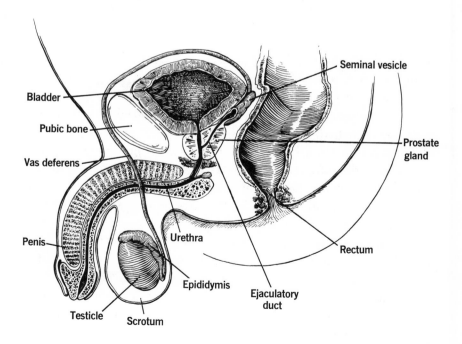

The Male Sex Organs

During ejaculation the muscles surrounding the base of the penis (the bulbocavernosus muscles and the ischiocavernosus muscles) contract powerfully and violently at 0.8 second intervals, and squirt the semen out of the penis with such force that it can travel a distance of one to two feet. The process of emission and ejaculation is an elegant, precisely orchestrated event, all coordinated via the sympathetic nerves coming from the mid-level of the spinal cord. This is an entirely different system of nerves from those that cause the blood vessels of the penis to open up and the penis to become erect.

Thus, emission is the contraction of the internal sex muscles to collect the various components of the ejaculate and place them in the bulb of the urethra. Ejaculation is the contraction of the external sex muscles, which squirt this fluid to the outside. Once emission occurs, it is impossible to delay ejaculation voluntarily.

The Brain Is the Most Important Sex Organ

Although the motor and sensory nerves of the penis orchestrate the intricate mechanical and electronic interplay of events that result in arousal and intercourse, we should not forget that the most important sex organ of all is the brain. The brain has been very intricately mapped for speech areas, hearing, vision, athletic coordination, breathing, vomiting, hiccuping, nausea, and for the specific regions that allow us to move just about every muscle in the body. We even know about the primitive area of the brain, the hypothalamus, that controls the interplay of hormonal events in the female's menstrual cycle and, in the male, the steady release of neurotransmitters that stimulate the testicles to make hormones and sperm. But we do not have a very clear representation of what specific site in the brain is responsible for sexual arousal, erection, and ejaculation.

In general, sexual arousal is a diffuse phenomenon in the brain that has its greatest activity in some of the primitive lower regions, but which also has modifying influences from higher cortical areas. Stimulation of a variety of regions has been able to produce erections repeatedly in monkeys. These are all part of a primitive portion of the brain located underneath the cerebral cortex (where thinking occurs), called the limbic system. Humans have the most complex brain of all animals, and thus have a much greater amount of cerebral complexity, which can both inhibit and excite these lower regions that affect sexuality. Sex in humans thus is not a simple primitive reflex response, but can be modified greatly by the most complex areas of the brain. Although erection is not under voluntary control, it is profoundly influenced nonetheless by a man's thoughts and whole conscious reflection about himself and his partner.

The Hydraulics of Erection

It is simple enough to understand that in humans erection is caused by the penis filling with blood, becoming engorged, distended, and thus rigid. In many other animals, including the whale, the bear, and the walrus, there is a bone called the os penis that provides most of the support and rigidity for intercourse. But the human mechanism of erection is more exquisitely refined than that of any other animal. For many years there was a controversy about just how it is that the penis fills with blood, what prevents all this blood from clotting during a prolonged erection, and why it is that in impotent men the penis does not fill up with blood sufficiently to cause it to get rigid.

It used to be thought that the penis became erect because the veins draining blood out of it closed off and trapped the arterial blood inside. There are some urologists even today who think this entrapment of blood is what causes erection. But modern experiments have dispelled that notion. If it were true that erection is caused by blood not draining out of the penis, then it would be simple enough for an impotent man to create an erection by putting a rubber band around the base of his penis. In fact, experiments like this have been performed, and all that happens is that the penis becomes black and blue and swollen, but no erection results.

We now know that erection occurs not because of any restriction of blood leaving the penis, but rather because of a tremendous increase in blood flowing *to* the penis. How does this occur? To study this question, experiments have been performed on cadavers in which tremendous amounts of fluid were pumped into the internal pudendal arteries (the arteries that directly supply the penis with blood). Despite infusion of tremendous volumes of fluid at rapid rates and with high pressures, erections could not be created. Yet in similar experiments, when fluid was pumped directly into the corpora cavernosa at flows of greater than four teaspoons per minute, erection did occur. Once the erection is initiated, it can be maintained with a much slower flow of only two teaspoons per minute. These cadaver experiments were then actually repeated on normal living male volunteers, with the same results. Thus erection is caused by a specific increase in blood flow to the corpora cavernosa of the penis. Once the corpora are distended, a smaller continual influx of blood is required to keep pace with the steady outflow. When the erection is over, the influx of blood reduces again to less than two teaspoons per minute, and the veins can then catch up with the arteries and allow the penis to drain so that it becomes limp.

It is not simply a matter of the penis being overfilled with blood, because no matter how much blood is pumped into the arteries supplying the penis, nothing very dramatic occurs except for blood going right back out again. What is required for erection to occur is that millions of tiny valves (frequently called polsters), which guard the entrance to the corpus cavernosum, open up, and allow a dramatic inflow of blood. Quite remarkably, it is sexual arousal that relaxes these valves so that the corpora can become engorged.

The erect penis has a pressure within it that is no greater than the standard blood pressure in all the arteries of the body. When the penis is not erect, this pressure never reaches the corpora. Thus all that is required for erection to occur is a relaxation of the penile valves so that the pressure maintained throughout the arterial system and the rest of the body is actually allowed to get into the penis.

Thus erection is a very precise and highly regulated event. Just the right amount of blood must flow in to allow a firm, rigid penis without painful overdistention. An intricately balanced system of microscopic valves open and close in response to our sexual thoughts, creating the erections that we often take for granted as a simple, dumb, animal response!

Males Compared to Females

The genital organs of men and women develop from identical structures. As a result of this common origin, there are basic similarities in the male and the female sexual apparatus. It is just as important for men to know what is happening in the female during intercourse as what is happening in the male.

There are basically two aspects of sex, erection and orgasm. Erection in the male is caused by the penis filling rapidly and inflating with blood in response to sexual arousal. During the equivalent event in females, the clitoris (which resembles a miniature version of the male penis located above the entrance to the vagina) also becomes engorged with blood. In the male, orgasm is triggered by continual stimulation of the glans (the tip of the penis) and the shaft; in the female, orgasm is triggered by stimulation of the clitoris. Orgasm involves the contraction of the same muscles in the woman as in the man, but in the woman there is no ejaculation of semen.

There are, of course, many obvious differences between the male and the female sexual systems, but it is important to understand that there is not as much physical difference between men and women as is commonly supposed. Such an understanding can go a long way toward preventing the sexual difficulties that can be caused by ignorance of the physical makeup of the opposite sex.

Changes in Erection and Orgasm with Age

Impotence is the biggest fear that any man has about his genitals. The scary thought that one evening in the heat of passion his penis will not become erect has worried most men at some time or other in their lives. In younger men an episode of impotence is usually entirely psychological and very transient; once a young man's anxiety about performance is overcome, his potency inevitably returns. But as men get somewhat older, and enter the late thirties, forties, and fifties, there is a slow, natural deterioration that can be very frightening.

When the male is in his late teens and early twenties, erections come on quickly, easily, and with the slightest provocation. Any period of sexual abstinence usually results in frequent wet dreams (also known as nocturnal emissions). On any evening it is not unusual for a young man to enter into a second or third episode of intercourse. The sexual appetite is powerful, and even a poor relationship, with a frank lack of interest in one's sexual partner, often does not get in the way of performance. But as early as the late twenties and progressively through the thirties, forties, and fifties, there is a gradual decline. This is not what we think of as impotence, and there is nothing that can be done about it. It is simply what males must expect to normally occur as they grow older.

There are seven basic changes to watch for. Although they are all signs of gradual deterioration in a man's sexual ability, many of them tend to be interpreted as benefits rather than hindrances, since they maximize sexual pleasure for both the man and his partner. First, it takes a little bit longer for sexual arousal to result in a good, firm erection. The young man in his late teens walking around with an erection so firm under his pants that it is embarrassing is a common occurrence. But it doesn't happen to the thirty year old. Even during sexual foreplay the sudden, firm pull that is ready before the pants are off, a frequent event with younger men, is not usually the case as they get older. This delay in erection in the older man forces him to engage in a longer period of foreplay with his partner, thus arousing her to a greater degree prior to penetration. Thus, although the slower erection is a sign of a gradual decline in the sexual response, it frequently results in better sex.

Second, the older men become, the longer it takes to reach orgasm, and the easier it is to delay or control ejaculation. Thus a young woman in her twenties who marries a man in his fifties may be under the impression that her husband has much greater sexual prowess than her previous twenty-year-old boyfriend, because her husband can go so much longer before he finally ejaculates. Actually, this delay in orgasm, which may result in heightened sexual pleasure, is just another sign of the inevitable deterioration that takes place with age.

Third, the orgasm becomes briefer and briefer every year, and fourth, the force of expulsion of the semen from the penis also decreases. Fifth, the volume of the ejaculate gets smaller and smaller with age. Sixth, as a man gets older he finds that he loses his erection very rapidly after orgasm has occurred, whereas in a young man it takes a little while for the erection to subside.

The seventh and possibly most disturbing aspect of this normal deterioration of sexual response is a lengthening of what we call the refractory period. In men (in marked contrast to women), it is impossible after orgasm for another erection or another episode of intercourse to occur until a certain period of time has passed. In a young man in his late teens the refractory period can be as brief as twenty minutes. But as he grows older the refractory period gets longer and longer. In women, no matter what the age, it usually takes longer to get aroused, but once aroused to the point of orgasm she is capable of heightened excitability and multiple orgasms if sexual stimulation is continued. But once the male has his orgasm he has no choice but to wait around until his refractory period is over.

It is not difficult to understand how this decline in sexual response can make a man so anxious about his performance that he may become totally unable to get any erections at all. He bases this anxiety on a mistaken notion that this decrease in his physiological functions means that it is all over for him. In truth, this is not at all the case. If he can accept this inevitable change in his normal processes, then this fear of not being able to perform should no longer make him so anxious that he cannot perform at all.

Some aspects of the decline in sexual response can actually be used to great advantage by allowing the female more foreplay and a longer duration of intercourse with a greater chance of having multiple orgasms. Thus the prolongation of sexual activity brought about by a man's decreasing ability to get an erection and to reach a quick orgasm as he gets older has its positive aspects.

2

Erections During Sleep

The Penis During Sleep

It may come as a surprise to most men to learn that they have at least five full unused erections, each lasting as long as thirty minutes, every night during their sleep from infancy to old age. Even men who for psychological reasons can't obtain erections when they want to have sex will repeatedly have them while they're sleeping. You would think that such a startling phenomenon would have been known down through history just as surely as the observation that sexual intercourse leads to pregnancy and that castration destroys a man's interest in sex. But for some reason no one was aware of this phenomenon until about 1945, when several German investigators described it in an obscure scientific journal read by very few doctors. These Germans observed many subjects while sleeping and found that erections occurred regularly every eighty-four minutes and had an average duration of twenty-five minutes.

About ten years later, scientists discovered that there is a phase of sleeping, occurring at ninety-minute intervals and lasting about half an hour, during which the sleeper's eyes move back and forth at a tremendous pace almost as though viewing some sort of movie taking place inside the brain. By waking subjects during various phases of their sleep it was discovered that it is during this rapid eye movement sleep (REM sleep) that dreaming occurs. If the subject is awakened during REM sleep, he can vividly remember his dream. However, if he is awakened within a minute after the REM phase ends, he can recall his dream only vaguely. If he is awakened five minutes after REM sleep has ended, he cannot remember any dreams at all.

Interestingly, erections occur during almost the entirety of our dreaming time, even though most of the time the dreams are in no way erotic. In other words, it is not as though we are having regular erotic dreams five times a night.

Almost all men at one time or other in their lives have difficulty obtaining an erection when they want to have intercourse with their partner. Sometimes this impotence is not temporary and becomes a great source of distress. The reason it is important to know about erections during sleep is that the knowledge merely can be used to determine whether the impotent man is suffering from psychological stress that will go away with counseling, or whether he has a physical problem.

The man who has only a psychological inhibition preventing him from becoming erect will have normal, maximum, firm erections every night while he sleeps no matter how impotent he may be while he is awake. However, the patient with a serious physical cause of his impotence will either have no erections during sleep or very poor or infrequent erections. Thus, it behooves us to understand fully the process of the erections men have during sleep.

Another reason to study nocturnal erections is to determine whether the gradual decline in sexual response as men get older is due to a declining psychological interest in sex or whether it is physical and unavoidable. Scientists have studied nightly erections (known as nocturnal penile tumescence or NPT) with such exactness that they now know precisely what degree of deterioration of erectile capability can be expected from all men as they get older. Let's look at the details of these scientific studies so that we can also understand just how much males can expect from their penises as they get older.

What Erections During Sleep Can Tell You

Studying erections during sleep is essentially just like taking an overnight electrocardiogram of the penis. An electrode in the form of a slender wire (called a mercury strain-gauge electrode) is placed around the penis before the patient goes to sleep. As the penis becomes erect, its circumference increases, causing this wire sensor to stretch. The stretching is measured and graphed. The next morning the doctor simply looks at the graph coming off the machine as if it were an electrocardiogram and finds out how many times the patient had an erection during the night, how long they lasted, and how large they were.

Since penises exist in many different sizes, an increase in circumference that would be sufficient to indicate a good, firm erection in the case of one man might not indicate a good erection in that of another. If the circumference of the penis increases by more than one inch, the erection is usually firm enough to permit good penetration of the vagina. If there is an increase of less than one inch in circumference, the erection will usually be soft, bendable, and inadequate for sex. Modern equipment for measuring these differences is so sensitive that doctors have no difficulty characterizing and quantifying in great detail the sufficiency of nocturnal erections.

In the sophisticated sex research laboratories at Baylor University in Houston, subjects slept with electrodes attached to their scalps and their penises so that erection (NPT) and dreaming could be studied simultaneously. This way it was possible to find out whether the decline in sexual ability that occurs as men get older is caused by a decline in the brain's ability to stimulate the penis (as would be shown by a decline in REM sleep time), or whether it is a decline in the ability of the penis itself to respond to the brain's stimulation.

What these tests showed was that the total amount of REM sleep time is fairly constant as one gets older, but the amount of REM erection time decreases dramatically. Thus it appears that the brain is not losing its ability to stimulate erections as one gets older, but that the whole penile apparatus is simply losing its ability to respond to the brain's stimulus.

Perhaps more important than the gradual decrease in the number of erections and the duration of individual erections is the fact that erections still occur with remarkable regularity as one gets older, most of them sufficiently firm to allow adequate intercourse. Thus, men of advanced age with no other problem may expect a slight slowing in their sexual performance, but they still should be able to have satisfying sex lives.

The Stamp Test

Luckily there is a simpler method for determining the presence of nightly erections, one that any man can use without having to consult a physician or go to the expense of attaching complicated electronic machinery to his penis. It is called the stamp test. This is how it works. Simply buy a roll of about six postage stamps from the post office and wrap them firmly around your penis near the base before going to sleep at night. Use Scotch tape at each end of the roll to hold the stamps in place. Depending upon the penis's size, as few as three or as many as six stamps may be required. During the night, the increase in diameter of the penis during erection will be sufficient to break this stamp collar along one of the perforations. If the stamps are torn, but not along the perforations, it simply means that while you tossed and turned the stamps got caught on something and were torn accidentally. This sort of tear does not indicate an erection. So, if you wake up in the morning and find the stamps lying on your bed, torn neatly along the perforations, you will know that you had a good erection while you slept.

There is a psychotherapeutic benefit to this test as well. Doctors have found that many men with psychologically induced impotence are cured overnight once they find out that their impotence is indeed only psychological. As soon as they wake up and find that the stamps have broken neatly along the perforation, indicating that they had normal erections during the night, their confidence is renewed. When the next opportunity for intercourse takes place, their penis doesn't fail them.

3

Hormones and Sex

Hormones and Sexual Desire

Many people have the mistaken notion that the male hormone (testosterone) stimulates the sexual urge in men, and that female hormones (estrogen and progesterone) stimulate the sexual urge in women. In actuality it is the male hormone that stimulates the sex drive in both men and women. Men make about ten times more male hormone than females, and females make about ten times more female hormone than males. But we all make both male and female hormones.

In the past, some male homosexuals were given large doses of testosterone in an effort to change their sexual preferences and make them more "manly" in their desires. The only change was that their libido, or sex drive, increased; their homosexuality remained. When females are given large doses of female hormones, for whatever medical reason, their libido is unchanged. Yet when you give male hormones to women, for whatever medical reason, the libido increases dramatically. Thus, the male hormone, testosterone, has no effect on sexual preference and does not distinguish between men and women in stimulating sexual interest.

Although the female hormones have no effect on a woman's sexuality, they have a profound effect on her breasts, the lining of her reproductive organs, and the menstrual cycle. While the male hormone is responsible for a woman's sexuality, it can be detrimental to her fertility unless present in only small amounts. Male hormone suppresses the ovary's sensitivity to the stimulatory effects of hormones coming from the brain and pituitary, so that it produces less female hormone, thus inhibiting ovulation.

Although giving male hormone to the female enhances her libido, giving female hormone to the male will suppress his libido. One of the major reasons for this is that the female hormone will inhibit the man's brain from stimulating his testicles to make male hormone. It might seem from this that birth control pills (which are simply female hormones) would suppress a woman's production of male hormone also and thus decrease her libido. But that is not the case, since most of a woman's male hormone is not produced by the ovary, but rather by the adrenal gland, which is located high in the abdomen just above the kidney. Birth control pills affect the ovaries, leaving the production of testosterone by the adrenal gland unchanged. This is also why when a woman goes through her change of life, and the ovaries shrivel up and disappear, she retains her sexual drive. The hormones responsible for her sexual drive have little to do with her fertility or her reproductive apparatus. Her male hormone, testosterone, is her hormone of sexuality, and it continues to be produced for her whole life.

Man is the only being in the entire animal kingdom whose desire for sex is so remarkably separate from the function of reproduction. In all other animals, the inclination to have sex only occurs several days prior to the female's ovulation, or just at the time when sex is likely to lead to conception. It is only in humans that the inclination to have sex occurs at any time of the month or year. The reason for this dramatic difference between man and all other animals is that in other animals the female's sex desire is created by the female hormones, which increase just prior to ovulation. In the female of all other species the same hormones that are preparing the womb with a rich lining to nourish the egg and are stimulating the ovary to release the egg are also the hormones that stimulate her interest in having sex. Thus female animals are likely to desire sex only at the moment the egg is about to be ovulated. But in human females, the buildup of the lining of the womb and ovulation have nothing to do with sexual desire. It is the male hormone, which is constantly and steadily produced by the woman's adrenal gland, that is responsible for her libido.

Although a woman produces about as much male hormone from her adrenal gland as a man does, her brain requires a smaller amount of it than does his to create an adequate libido. That is why the tiny amount of male hormone produced by the adrenal gland in both men and women is enough for the female. However, the male requires considerably more testosterone to stimulate his libido, which is why he needs his testicles, which pour out huge amounts of testosterone—ten times the amount produced by the female.

The effect of male hormones on the female was brought out very clearly to me last year when a couple came to my office, complaining of infertility. The husband was twenty-eight years old and his wife was twenty-six. They had already had one child, a girl, and had been trying to have their second for the past seventeen months without success. The wife had gone to her local doctor one day and happened to mention that she was feeling tired. Of course that would certainly be understandable of a woman with a one-year-old toddler running around. But her doctor did something quite incredible and gave her a huge shot of testosterone. Immediately thereafter she had a tremendous increase in her libido, but her menstrual periods had been irregular ever since. While the testosterone had tremendously boosted her sex drive, it had badly suppressed the ability of her ovaries to make female hormones and to ovulate.

By this point you may begin to worry that perhaps sex is not so much an expression of a mental desire as it is simply a chemical reaction. The way we have been talking, it may sound as though the desire to have sex is regulated purely by testosterone. It all seems rather dull and chemical. But fortunately it is not that simple. Testosterone creates a basic urge, a libido, which seems to be a motor that is running all the time in neutral, ready to go into drive when we are aroused sexually. But that is all it is. The brain (and by that I don't mean simply the primitive area of the brain that regulates hormone production, but rather the higher centers of thought in the brain) is still the most important sex organ. Without testosterone, the higher regions in our brain may not be very interested in sex, but testosterone does not determine when we want it or with whom we want it.

What is it that testosterone does, how does it drive the libido, how much help is it in successful sexual intercourse, and what effects does it have on the body other than simply creating the desire for sex? It is important for us to know exactly what testosterone does, because if it is some sort of miracle hormone that endows men and women with sexual desire and ability, perhaps it would have a role in treating impotence and frigidity.

Testosterone and Sexual Ability

First, we should make it clear that testosterone does not endow the male with his ability to have erections. Men are quite capable of having erections without male hormone. In fact, little boys have erections quite frequently, as any parent can tell you. Most men who complain of impotence or of a declining ability to have successful sexual relations are really complaining that they cannot become erect, or that their erections are too soft for vaginal penetration. Very often this is incorrectly blamed on a decline in testosterone production with age. This is but one of the many staggering misconceptions about testosterone and sexual ability. The level of male hormone does not significantly decline as men get older. If there is any such thing as a male menopause, it is not related to a decline in hormone production. Men throughout their fifties, sixties, and seventies continue to produce essentially the same amount of hormone that they were producing in their late teens and twenties. In fact, if a man's hormone levels really declined as he got older, he would not complain about an inability to obtain an erection, because he would not care. Since a normal testosterone level is necessary to maintain a baseline libido, a man whose testosterone production had declined would have little concern about his inability to obtain an erection.

Erections seem to be controlled automatically and involuntarily by the brain. A man cannot simply will an erection when he wants one. It must come on automatically as a result of sexual arousal, and is not dependent on male hormone or willpower. Hormones only affect the desire for sex, not the ability to carry it out.

But male hormone does have profound physical effects on the male body, in addition to the overall stimulation of sexual desire. We are all familiar with the effects of puberty, as males change from little boys to men—the deepening of the voice, the growth of a beard and body hair, the development of pubic hair, the elongation and enlargement of the penis, the strengthening of the musculature, and even the sudden growth spurt of adolescence, not to mention the increased oiliness of the skin. All of these effects of testosterone on the male body are called secondary sex characteristics. Without testosterone men would not have them. Even baldness requires testosterone. That does not mean that bald men have more testosterone than men who have kept their hair, but just that those men with a genetic predisposition to baldness cannot become bald unless they also have testosterone. Men who have no testicles do not go bald, just as most women do not.

Eunuchs—What Is It Like Without Testosterone?

In ancient days, boys who were destined to become servants in a harem were castrated before puberty, thus becoming eunuchs. They never went through adolescence or puberty, they retained the high-pitched voice of childhood, developed no beard, and maintained a boyish, infantile-sized penis. These eunuchs never under-went the profound adolescent growth spurt that boys normally have at around age twelve; they did eventually reach normal height, but it took much longer. Their muscle mass did not in-crease, and the growing plate in their bones never closed. They had long, spindly arms with thin muscles, very little body hair, and no beard, but they had very thick and beautiful hair on their heads and they never became bald. And, even though they were capable of having erections, they had no interest in using them.

What about castration after puberty? Once the male has formed all of the secondary sex characteristics, does he continue to need testosterone in order to maintain them? The interesting fact is that men who are castrated after they achieve puberty retain just about all of their secondary sex characteristics. Their voice remains deep, their muscle mass does not thin out, they do not get shorter, their penis remains essentially the same length, and they even retain their pubic hair. Despite the fact that they have no testicles and do not make testosterone in any quantity greater than females do, they continue to look like normal men.

But does a castrated man retain his interest in sex, or does it decline as soon as his testosterone is gone? Interestingly, there is a wide variation, but most castrated men do retain their libido for a certain period of time. It tends to diminish gradually, and eventually in most cases the desire for sex goes away completely. But this decline is not altogether sudden, and it is not completely predictable. The effects of testosterone on the brain, causing a desire for sex, may last for a while even after the hormone is gone. The intensity of the libido may be diminished rather quickly, but if the intensity of mental desire for sex is strong enough, at least for a period of time, it can overcome the lack of the hormone. Eventually, however, without hormones sexual desire disappears.

Some men are only part eunuch. They may not realize that their puberty was mediocre because of poorly functioning testi-cles, which made only a small amount of testosterone. These men don't have that complete lack of interest in sex that characterizes eunuchs. They may even be married and trying to have children before they realize that things are not quite right. Here is a typical example.

A twenty-eight-year-old man and his wife came to see me with fertility problems. The man was able to ejaculate only a small specimen, which had no sperm in it. He had very small testicles, sparse pubic hair, and he rarely had to shave. He had gone through puberty at eleven years of age, and he seemed to be having adequate sex with his wife. He had no idea that there was anything wrong with him, yet he was producing only half of the normal amount of testosterone. His pituitary hormones were very high, indicating that his body was working as hard as possible to make his testicles produce as much testosterone as possible. His sex chromosomes, instead of having the normal XY male pattern, had an XXY pattern, a condition known as Klinefelter's syndrome. He was a normal, intelligent man in every other way, and he thought that he had gone through puberty normally. What he didn't realize was that his level of sex hormone was low, and the slightest emotional disturbance was enough to turn off completely his already shallow libido.

As soon as I placed him on testosterone injections every two weeks in an effort to bring his male hormone level up to normal, his beard became thicker, his voice became deeper, he developed a dramatic increase in his sexual desire, and his penile length even increased. Testosterone shots helped him to complete the puberty that he had only partially and inadequately gone through seventeen years earlier.

This patient, like other partial eunuchs undergoing replacement injections of testosterone, was much more dependent on the hormone for his moods and sex drive from day to day than normal men. Twelve days after each injection he would begin to get crabby, his mood would become depressed, and his sexual desire would decrease. This correlated closely with the decline in the level of hormone that usually occurs twelve days after an injection. Then, as soon as he had the injection again, his sex drive would increase and he would become more cheerful and optimistic.

The most dramatic example of this turning on and turning

off of sexual desire with testosterone injections was a patient upon whom we performed the first testicle transplant. He had been born without any testicles and would have been a complete eunuch except that his doctors began giving him testosterone injections at age eighteen to create an artificial puberty. Although this caused his beard to grow, his penis to lengthen, and gave him a sex drive, these effects were quite volatile. Immediately after an injection he would have a very intense desire for sex, but when the level of hormone dropped a week and a half after the injection, his sex drive would go away just as rapidly as it had come, and he would become depressed. It was only after he received a successful transplant of one of his twin brother's testicles that his sex drive and his temperament became more even.

This patient reports that prior to having his own testicle, he felt that his sex drive was dependent upon those injections. He felt that his mind had very little to do with the intense need for sex that he felt shortly after the injection. Yet a week or so later, when the level of testosterone in his system was dropping, he had very little interest in sex. This up-and-down sex drive, purely dependent upon chemicals, diminished the spontaneity and active mental participation in sex that characterizes humans. Once he had his own normal testicle with a more constant level of testosterone, he felt that he was participating more actively in his sex interest, and was not simply a body being flogged around by chemicals surging within his system beyond his control.

Is Sex Chemical?

There is obviously much that is unknown about the mysterious effects of the male hormone, testosterone, on male sexuality. Interestingly, doctors know more about the sex life of rats and how testosterone affects it than they do about humans'. But scientists feel that much of this information also applies to man. So let's review a little bit about how testosterone affects the male rat's sex life and reflect on what this may mean for humans.

In the rat, male sexual behavior is quantitatively related to the amount of male hormone. Castration of the rat results in an immediate and progressive decline in the likelihood of ejaculatory behavior. Testosterone disappears from the circulation within a few hours after castration, but the sexual behavior that was programmed by testosterone continues on in one form or another for days, weeks, months, and sometimes even years, though in a diminished fashion. After all sexual behavior has completely stopped in the castrated rat, giving him testosterone injections will fully reinstate it. The male rat may continue to mount the female and insert his penis, but the ability to ejaculate and achieve orgasm in the absence of testosterone is the first sexual function to go. Sexual behavior thus declines in sequence rather than all at once, and there is a considerable time lag between castration and the final extinction of all sexual behavior. This time lag has been noted in every species studied to date.

The key question raised by such studies is whether there is any relationship between the different amounts of testosterone in different men and their degree of sexual interest and ability. To put it in a crude way, one might ask whether men with higher testosterone production are better lovers.

The amount of testosterone required to maintain sexual behavior is considerably less than the normal circulating level in most men, which means that there is normally much more testosterone in their system (except for eunuchs or partial eunuchs) than they require to maintain a good sex life. Furthermore, as long as the testosterone level is within a normal range, there is no correlation between the variation in hormone level in normal men at any particular time and the amount of sex they desire. There seems to be a certain minimal amount of testosterone necessary to engender a strong libido. Once that minimal amount is achieved, it requires huge increases caused by shots or external administration to make any discernible difference in sexual desire. Thus, men with naturally higher testosterone production are not necessarily more interested in sex.

The next inescapable question is whether impotence and lack

of sexual interest are caused by a decreased amount of testosterone, or whether increasing the amount of testosterone can correct these conditions. If we look at large numbers of experimental rats, we will occasionally come across an otherwise healthy rat that simply does not want to have sex. Animal breeders call this type of rat a "noncopulator." Studies of these noncopulating rats show that they have slightly lower levels of testosterone than normal rats, but much higher levels of testosterone than are usually required by normal rats to have sexual interest. Scientists have concluded therefore that an impotent rat has two separate problems. Certainly its level of testosterone is somewhat low, but not low enough to directly cause impotence. The major problem is that this impotent rat has a low sensitivity to the effect of testosterone. That brings up the whole question of where testosterone acts and how it stimulates interest in sex. Does testosterone act directly on the brain to get the sexual apparatus in gear, or does it act specifically on the sex organs, creating the urge within them for sexual release?

It is now clear that the major effect of testosterone in terms of libido is on the brain, and in animals scientists have rather specifically located that region of the brain where testosterone has this sex-stimulating effect. By stimulating this specific area of the brain in rats, it is possible to restore their sexual function *even after they have been castrated.* The brain receives general libido encouragement from testosterone, but specific sexual arousal comes not from testosterone but from the brain's own storehouse of experience in life. The brain is not chemically turned on and off by normal fluctuations in testosterone. Once an adequate level of circulating testosterone has been established, the degree of sexual desire is no longer hormonal. Rather, the fluctuations of sexual desire are dependent upon the brain's total range of prior experience.

Several years ago there was a study that indicated that homosexual men had lower testosterone levels than heterosexual males. The investigators (who were rather prominent in their field) therefore suggested that homosexuality had a hormonal basis.

Nothing could be more naïve or further from the truth. Several more recent, carefully controlled studies have failed to show any difference in the level of testosterone in homosexual males as compared to heterosexual males. Neither men with low testosterone levels nor women with high testosterone levels become homosexuals. Homosexuality is not caused by hormones; rather, it is an intellectual and emotional orientation of sexual preference, unrelated to any hormonal imbalance in adulthood. Testosterone stimulates interest in sex, but it has no effect on sexual preference.

The unisexuality of the human sexual response to hormones is unique in the animal kingdom. The human sex drive, from a hormonal point of view, is neither male nor female but rather an undifferentiated basic urge created by a single hormone, testosterone. The differences in sexual desire, not only from the point of view of gender choice and choosing a mate, but also the entire emotional-intellectual network of lovemaking in humans, are left up to the brain. In that respect, humans are quite emancipated from their animal secretions, compared to all other members of the biological world. The content of erotic inclination in the human species is not controlled by the sex hormones at all, but rather by the brain, which is our most important sex organ.

Hormones and Sex Crimes

I recently met an endocrinologist from England who told me about a frightening case involving a teenage boy who had been born without testicles, and who had not gone through puberty until he was put on testosterone injections at age sixteen. It is not clear whether the dose of testosterone was excessive, but the boy —who had previously been quiet and docile—went through an incredibly violent puberty, with the result that he murdered a little girl in a sexual assault. This case brings up the question of whether testosterone may cause criminal sexual behavior, and whether treatment to lower the testosterone level might be used to cure or alleviate criminal sex tendencies.

Psychiatrists who have studied criminal sex offenders find that all of these men tend to report a constant feeling of insatiable sexual desire, despite having a normal level of testosterone. These men are much more sensitive to the normal male amount of testosterone, so that it creates in them an uncontrollable sexual rage. Interestingly, women almost never commit sex crimes. It seems that the amount of testosterone in women is just sufficient to create a normal libido, but is low enough to prevent any compulsive, criminal sexual urge. It seems that you need the extra amount of testosterone that men normally have in order to be compelled toward committing sex crimes.

For one reason or another, sex offenders cannot mentally control their sexual appetite except by acting it out in antisocial ways. To what extent is it their hormones, and to what extent their psychological makeup, that drives them to such criminal acts as rape, child molesting, or exhibitionism?

Studies at Johns Hopkins University in Baltimore and the University of Texas in Galveston have shown that lowering the production of testosterone in these sex offenders relieves their insatiable desire so they no longer feel the need to commit sex crimes. The scientific studies of these offenders tell much about how hormones can affect normal as well as abnormal sexual activity.

Men who feel the compulsion to commit sex crimes have a condition which psychiatrists call paraphilia. Paraphiliacs usually cannot have normal sexual activity, and erotic pleasure occurs only when their fantasies are enacted precisely. Behavior therapists have tried aversion therapy as a treatment. For example, an electric shock is applied to such a patient whenever he reports having an erotic thought about children or about rape. But this approach has been completely unsuccessful in correcting the deviant sexual impulses that seem to be totally beyond their conscious will.

However, giving sex offenders the female hormone Depo-Provera (which completely inhibits the production of male hormone) relieves their sexual urges, and they no longer commit these criminal offenses while they are on the medication. This hormone does not cause men to become feminized in appearance or to have a homosexual sex preference. All it does is inhibit their brain from releasing the factor that stimulates the testicles to make testosterone. As soon as male hormone production ceases, so do the deviant sexual cravings. Most of these patients report tremendous relief from the criminal sexual compulsions over which they otherwise have no control.

Professor John Money from Johns Hopkins and Professor Paul Walker from the University of Texas have pioneered the use of Depo-Provera to abolish this testosterone-dependent desire without which the criminal act cannot easily occur. Professors Money and Walker insistently point out that sex offenders do not have an abnormally high amount of testosterone; rather, a normal amount of male hormone simply allows the abnormal mental condition to express itself. They feel that the problem of these criminals dates back to early childhood and faulty sex modeling. They state in their report: "The sex offender behaves as though sexual activity with an adult member of the opposite sex is somehow or other cheap, dirty, illegal, and immoral. Their behavior implies an ethic of a willing partner as a cheap whore and therefore undesirable. The only appropriate sexual partner becomes the innocent and pure partner—the unwilling, the unsuspecting, or the child." Dr. Walker particularly admonishes our society to avoid instilling such an ethic into children at an early age.

But once the criminal mind has been established, the only successful therapy has been hormonal. Approximately 400 mg. of Depo-Provera is injected once a week for at least six months. The goal of the therapy is to eliminate all erotic desire. The patients report a complete vacation from sexual imagery and desire. During this time, psychotherapy is instituted in an attempt to change the orientation of the patient. Otherwise, when he stops taking the medication, the urge toward criminal sexual behavior will assuredly return. The patients do not complain about the loss of sexual interest caused by the Depo-Provera shots, but rather report a sense of relief from their otherwise intrusive sexual compulsion.

Testosterone Injections and Impotence

If giving a drug like Depo-Provera to stop testosterone production can help sex criminals get over their uncontrollable libido, can the opposite work? That is, can impotent men be treated with testosterone supplements to improve their sexual functioning or their ability to get and maintain an erection adequate for intercourse? Many studies have now demonstrated that the impotent male, i.e., the man who either cannot get an erection or whose sexual interest has declined, rarely has a low testosterone level. There are a few cases where this is a problem, but the overwhelming majority of impotent men, even older ones, have normal levels of sex hormones. Even so, can giving an extra amount of testosterone, by injection or by pill, in some way give such men that extra boost they may need?

The notion that there might be a simple aphrodisiac that can cure impotence dates back thousands of years. Ground rhinoceros horn was (and in some countries still is) considered such a sure cure for failing sexual ability that this animal was hunted almost to extinction. Even today there are those who think that eating oysters may help. And a similar notion is being pumped into the heads of doctors by aggressive drug companies, whose advertisements promote the treatment of impotence with hormone shots or pills.

This erroneous notion that testosterone can cure impotence has spread far. I recently read in a newspaper advice column a letter from a woman who complained that her sex life had turned sour because her husband, at age fifty-two, could no longer get an erection. The columnist replied that one-third of sexually impotent men suffered from a hormone deficiency, and that almost all of them were able to resume normal sexual activity after being treated with testosterone—a well-intentioned but entirely false piece of information. Numerous scientific studies have demonstrated that most men suffering from impotence have completely normal levels of testosterone. If the husband wanted to have sex but was unable to have an erection, there is no physical way that a lack of testosterone could explain such symptoms. A lack of testosterone could only explain a loss of interest in having sex and a diminished libido.

The fact is that wherever they turn, doctors are bombarded with advertising implying that testosterone will cure impotence. Innuendo after innuendo in some of the most clever advertising ever directed at physicians tries to entice them into prescribing testosterone for their impotent patients. It is not the makers of the injectable testosterone that are doing most of this advertising—the profit margin with injectable testosterone is very low—but the manufacturers of the highly profitable chemical derivatives of testosterone, such as Halotestin and methyltestosterone, which can be taken as a pill instead of a shot. Yet the injectable testosterone is the only form of the hormone that can be administered with maximum safety and effectiveness, even to those patients who truly need testosterone replacement. The hormone testosterone is destroyed by the stomach juices and therefore cannot be taken as a pill. It has to be given as an injection. The pill forms are chemicals similar to testosterone that have been designed to resist stomach acids. Yet all of these pill versions are very weak in their actions compared to natural testosterone, and when administered in doses large enough to have an effect, they have an unacceptably high level of liver toxicity.

The drug companies making these oral preparations send advertisements to urologists and endocrinologists with a spectacular Madison Avenue approach. One drug company has a beautiful picture of a handsome man who looks around thirty-five years old staring into space, wondering something very deep, with a caption saying "He's impotent due to androgen deficiency. What do you prescribe?" The advertisement never mentions how rare it is for androgen deficiency to be the cause of impotence. In another advertisement from a different drug company there is a picture of a young man on the left and an older man (presumably the same man many years later) on the right with graying hair and a beard. The quotation between their faces says, "Does aging affect androgen production?" It leaves the casual reader with the notion that androgens cure impotent men. Then on the right in huge, bold letters is the brand name displayed as though it were the final answer. This advertisement fails to point out that even in rare conditions where testosterone production is deficient, despite the convenience of this pill form, it has more side effects and is less potent than the cheaper natural testosterone that has been available for the past thirty years.

If a man is suffering from psychological impotence, a shot of testosterone can sometimes boost his libido to the point where he may forget his inhibitions because his sexual urge is so intense. His confidence may be temporarily restored, but usually the increased libido caused by the injection results only in increased frustration for the impotent man. There are better methods of dealing with the inhibitions that are preventing him from getting successful erections. If his problem is organic, a surgical implant is the only chance he has for regaining normal erections (see Chapter 7). A testosterone injection will only heighten his sense of frustration by exaggerating his libido and do nothing for his ability to maintain an erection.

A seventy-two-year-old man I saw last year exemplifies the damage that can be done by the indiscriminate prescribing of testosterone. This man had lost his wife several years before and now was in love with a sixty-year-old woman. His son had recently died and he was very depressed. He was complaining of an intermittent inability to obtain erections with his new partner, and even when he could get an erection, it frequently was too soft for intercourse. A year before, a doctor had placed him on testosterone pills (Halotestin) three times a day. He was afraid to stop taking them because of the fear that if he did so, even his occasional erections would cease. He was under the impression that the only reason he could have sex at all was the fact that he was taking the testosterone pills.

We measured the hormone levels in his blood, something which had not been done before he was indiscriminately given Halotestin. I found that the testosterone level was extremely low because the weak testosterone pill was suppressing his pituitary gland, which would normally stimulate testosterone production. Thus, because of the pills he was taking, his own *natural* testosterone was very low. In a sense he was "hooked" on the pills, which in themselves were too weak to be very helpful. I immediately took him off the medication, and several months later his testosterone returned to normal levels.

Then we returned to the real cause of his impotence, which was psychological. After tests demonstrated that he was able to obtain normal erections four or five times every night during his sleep, he realized that there was nothing physically wrong, and this renewed confidence resulted in a rather dramatic return of potency. He is no longer on testosterone pills, he has a better, clearer view of himself and his sexual relationship with his mate, and he is no longer impotent.

There are some people who ill-advisedly take testosterone supplements for reasons totally unrelated to their potency. As you recall, when a young boy begins to go through puberty—a phenomenon entirely mediated by the sudden production of testosterone at about age twelve—he undergoes a sudden growth spurt and an increase in muscular development that his female counterpart does not experience. Aside from causing the development of pubic hear and a beard and deepening the voice, testosterone has a side effect that could be considered beneficial to many athletes, namely increasing their muscular development. When given to adults in excess amounts, testosterone can increase the size and power of their muscles. In addition, testosterone is known to bolster the production of red blood cells and thus enhance the body's utilization of oxygen. For these reasons the use of testosterone has become widespread in athletics.

There is a tremendous amount of pressure on all athletes to achieve and to be number one. It has been alleged that even in the Olympics a large percentage of the shot put, discus, and weight-lifting athletes used testosterone (commonly referred to as steroids) to increase their muscular power. Even more scary is that it is being used by female athletes to give them an advantage in muscular development for women's competitive sports requiring great strength. Athletes are very impressed by the ability of testosterone, either pills or injections, to improve their strength and performance, but most are not aware of the terrible risk of liver damage to those taking the pill versions of testosterone. In addition, few female athletes are aware of what testosterone does to their menstrual cycles and their ability to ovulate, and most male athletes are not aware that it suppresses their own testosterone and sperm production. But in this age of Super Bowl mentality, the athlete with the biggest muscles often wins the largest purse, and testosterone has certainly been an aid to many of them in obtaining that goal.

Questions often come up about whether the increased use of drugs in our society, from alcohol and marijuana to more dangerous drugs, affects potency or testosterone production. It is well known that males who are chronic alcoholics have a high risk of developing a condition called gynecomastia, in which they experience an abnormal enlargement of their breasts. One reason for this condition is that their damaged liver causes them to have a higher level of the female hormone estrogen, and this causes their breasts to become abnormally large. But equally important is the fact that alcohol also decreases the body's production of testosterone. In 1976 a very careful study by the Department of Medicine of the New York Medical College, published in the *New England Journal of Medicine*, demonstrated that when alcohol is given to normal male volunteers for periods of up to four weeks, there is a reduction in testosterone secretion that normally should come from the testicles, and the amount of testosterone circulating in the blood is diminished.

Are there similar adverse effects on testosterone production resulting from other drugs, such as heroin, marijuana, methadone, angel dust, speed, or any of the other popular cult drugs? On this matter, the studies are very conflicting. Regarding marijuana's effect, one study by a reputable author showed that sperm count was decreased but the testosterone level remained normal. A study by a different investigator showed that the sperm count remained normal but the testosterone level was decreased. All of these studies were performed with biased methodology, so we really don't have any clear-cut answer to whether marijuana or any of the other popular drugs have any effect on testosterone production, or potency.

However, the scientific evidence currently available in this field clearly demonstrates that an inability to obtain an erection is not a condition to be treated by indiscriminately prescribing testosterone. It is only a rare case of impotence that is truly caused by a hormonal deficiency, and souping up the system with extra testosterone will enhance the libido but not the ability, which could lead to even more frustration in the impotent man. Testosterone is only helpful to the man whose psychological problems are so mild that, with or without help, sooner or later his erections would return. Yet in the rare patient whose testicles do not produce an adequate amount of testosterone, the replacement of testosterone will dramatically improve his libido.

4

Sex and the Seasons

Humans are fortunate to enjoy an interest in sex throughout every month and season of the year. In most other animals, the male's testicles will grow and induce sexual desire only during a particular season, after which the testicles shrivel and sexual interest completely disappears for the rest of the year. A man who occasionally notices a downturn in sexual interest related to the momentary stress of a new life situation may gain some insight by learning what the animals experience. For humans, the ever-abundant, day-by-day, continuing desire to have sex is a unique gift that hardly any other animals enjoy.

During the winter a male bird's testicles actually shrivel up and become very tiny. However, as spring approaches he begins to feel something new happening again inside. He has no conscious control over this resurgence in sexual interest that returns automatically every year as the days begin to get longer. His testicles begin to grow every spring, producing massive amounts of male hormone responsible for his sex drive. At the same time, the female bird's ovaries begin to enlarge, and she too approaches her time of heat, when she will accept the male, receive his sperm, and use them to fertilize her eggs.

What happens in the spring that makes the bird's testicles suddenly begin to grow? Could it be that the warm weather and the pleasant days ahead in some way make the young male's fancy turn toward females? A romantic thought, but not true. It is not the warmth, it is not the rainfall, it is not the green grass, and it is not the budding flowers that cause his testicles to enlarge. It is simply the fact that the days are getting longer. The increasing day length stimulates a tiny structure in the middle of the bird's brain, called the pineal gland, to release a hormone that causes the hypothalamus to signal his testicles and thus awaken his whole reproductive apparatus. As the days get shorter in the fall, the pineal gland turns off and his testicles shrivel. But they lie in wait for the longer days of the following spring when they will once again be stimulated into action.

If you take a sexually inactive wintering bird and place it in a room where the light is kept on after it is dark outside, you can cause it to have a sudden sexual renaissance, long before spring arrives. In fact, chicken farmers have discovered that leaving a light in the henhouse will keep the hens producing eggs even as fall approaches, when egg production would normally end.

Hamsters, groundhogs, and some other animals go into a deep sleep called hibernation during the winter. During that time, their testicles shrink and they stop making testosterone and sperm. As spring approaches and the days get longer, their shriveled testicles suddenly begin to grow, just like the bird's. It is the message that the days are getting longer, given by the hamster's, or bird's eyes to its pineal gland that allows its testicles to grow.

If a male hamster were blinded, its testicles would shrink just as they do when winter approaches. A blind hamster has shriveled up, functionless testicles. But the process doesn't remain that simple. After a long period of time, a blinded hamster's pineal gland (despite getting no messages about daylight) will suddenly allow the testicles to grow anyway, and the blind hamster, after a long refractory period, regains its libido. But subsequently no matter what the season, its testicles will never shrivel again, despite the coming of winter. The only way its testicles could shrivel up again would be if its sight were restored, and it were then exposed again to the long days of summer followed by the short days of winter. This complex regulation of seasonal sexual ability in most animals is referred to by scientists as "photoperiodicity." It is regulated by the hormone melatonin produced by the pineal gland in the middle of the brain. In humans the pineal gland is only rudimentary (thank goodness), so our sexual ability does not seem to be influenced by either the length of the day or by the season.

But we humans have some variation of our own. It is known that human males have higher testosterone levels in the early morning than during the day. So we too in a small way undergo variation in sex hormone production, but it is according to the time of day. Furthermore, in large-scale population studies performed in France, the average sperm count was found to be highest in February and lowest in August. The average testosterone level of humans is highest in October, just four months prior to the peak in average sperm count. Although for all practical purposes male hormone and sperm production levels in humans are fairly even throughout the year, lacking the dramatic seasonal variations found in animals, nonetheless this slight but definite variation may be a vestige of our primitive heritage.

Why should there be this seasonal variation in sex in the animal kingdom? If baby birds were to be hatched in autumn during the flight south, there would be very few birds in the world. Animals need to be adapted temporally with their environment in order to multiply, and the simplest regulator is daylight. In certain animals there is a large variety of other cues that stimulate the primitive region of the brain to activate their reproductive apparatus. These cues include smell, vision, touch, temperature, hearing, and even the availability of certain nutrients in the diet. One or another of these cues will feed into the primitive region of an animal's brain and turn him on reproductively. But none of these sensations has been nearly so successful in the animal kingdom in stimulating reproductive organs as simply the length of day.

Let's look at some animals that normally just give up every-thing during the winter and hibernate. You may not have been aware of the fact that the reason the male groundhog goes into hibernation and slips into a deep sleep is that its testicles atrophy as the days get shorter. It is almost as if the groundhog decides that if he can't have sex, or at least a normal-sized pair of testicles to walk around with, there is just no point in carrying on any further. He finds himself a nice place to lie down and literally sleeps through the entire winter with his shriveled up testicles and his very low level of male hormone. If you were to remove his pineal gland, his testicles would not shrivel as autumn ap-proaches, and indeed he would not get sleepy or go into hiber-nation. He would retain his testicles and his alertness. Such a groundhog who had lost his pineal gland would want to have sex and reproduce all year round. As good as this sounds to us humans, it is very bad for the groundhog's survival, because some of its offspring would be born in winter and would have no chance to live.

An injection of testosterone given to a golden hamster or groundhog at the start of winter will prevent it from hibernating. Animals that are already hibernating will suddenly awaken upon the injection of testosterone pellets. Animals that are castrated during hibernation just do not wake up.

The change from seasonal sex and sleeping half the year toward the more continuous pleasure that we humans enjoy can be seen in hamsters that have been domesticated. Golden ham-sters used in the laboratory over a decade gradually require a longer duration of short periods of light to induce the testicles to shrivel. Whereas a decade ago these golden hamsters required less than four weeks for their testicles to shrivel, now they require at least twelve weeks of short days before they finally hibernate. Thus, laboratory animals gradually lose their sexual seasonability, because the survival of their offspring does not depend upon the time of year in which they are born. This has to make us wonder: If the survival of our species once again were to depend upon birth occurring in spring rather than winter, would the pineal gland (which is clearly present in the brain of all humans) suddenly become active and convert us once more into seasonal breeders?

There is a group of wild horses in the Pryor Mountains of Montana, called feral stallions, which were once domesticated animals. They were imported from England over a hundred years ago, but eventually they escaped and became wild. Most domesticated horses are not seasonal breeders, and the survival of their offspring does not depend upon being born in any particular season. But these once-domestic stallions of Montana now have their maximum testosterone levels in May, and that is the only month in which they mate. This ensures that the colt will be born the following spring, when it has a chance to survive in the wild. It is intriguing that these horses are interested in sex during any season while domestic, but that in the wild they have adapted by having sex only during the month of May.

Experiments with the rhesus monkey demonstrate that we primates indeed still *are* subject to the influence of light and darkness in the production of male hormone. If monkeys are placed in a room where the lights are on for twelve hours and then off for twelve, their testosterone levels go down when the lights are on and up when the lights are off. Thus, after twelve hours of darkness the rhesus monkey is producing the maximum amount of male hormone. That is why early in the morning in both monkeys and humans the male hormone level is at its maximum. It is simply a response in the most primitive manner to the lights going out. As day then wears on, the production of the male hormone also decreases, and by nightfall testosterone has reached its lowest level.

The thought that turning the lights out actually increases our sex hormone production might at first seem confusing, since in hamsters and birds it is a shorter day with decreased light that causes the testicles to atrophy and make less hormone. Yet in humans we find that turning out the lights, instead of causing the testicles to shrink, causes them to make more hormone. In that respect humans are more akin to other seasonal breeders such as the ram or the deer.

The ram's testicles only begin to grow and make male hormone as the days get shorter, which is quite the opposite of the
groundhog, whose testicles begin to shrivel when the days get
shorter. Any backpacker or hunter has seen how, as fall approaches, the bull moose, the buck, the stag, or the ram begins to
behave more and more irrationally and become increasingly interested in only one thing—sex. This brief seasonal burst of sexuality
is commonly known as rut.

The Asian elephant goes through the same phenomenon, but
it is called "musth." Ever since man first started to domesticate
male elephants thousands of years ago, it has been known that
once a year the bull becomes disobedient, aggressive, and extremely dangerous, often attempting to kill anybody who comes
within range. They must be completely chained for a month or so
for the safety of all around them.

In the male deer, or buck, rutting usually begins in September,
as days become shorter. The testicles begin to enlarge and make
male hormone. Just as testosterone causes humans to grow pubic
hair, it causes the male deer or moose to grow antlers. Only the
older and larger stags who carry the biggest antlers are able to
hold harems of females. If the antlers are cut off an otherwise
sexually successful stag, its behavior begins to fall apart and it is
no longer as able to hold its harem, even though it may have been
highly successful during the rut of the preceding year (and may
once again be successful in the following year when it grows new
antlers). As the end of November approaches and mating is completed, the testosterone level once again begins to drop, and the
male deer or moose becomes uninterested in sex for the rest of
the winter.

Sheep farmers who want to increase their herds have learned
that if they expose their breeding rams to short days with only
eight hours of light and sixteen hours of darkness during the
otherwise nonbreeding summer season, the ram's daily sperm production rises dramatically and the pregnancy rate doubles. In
humans, the vestige of the effect of darkness on sexuality is still
apparent. The testosterone level is always highest before the sun
rises, and then goes down with daylight. It is likely that this

fluctuation of the hormones, and the slighter seasonal fluctuation, are both vestiges of prehistoric man's greater susceptibility to natural forces. In those times humans, like other animals, probably bred at the time of year most likely to cause birth during clement weather. But the most important thing is that humans are no longer dependent on either hormonal fluctuations or changes in season for their sexual desire.

PART TWO
What Can Go Wrong

5

Perils of the Penis*

Most men tend to regard their genitals very protectively, and with good reason. The male genitalia are so incredibly exposed to potential injury or disease that all men have learned quite justifiably to regard them as their privates. There are many common perils of the penis that men need to be aware of in order to avoid them. But there are also some bizarre circumstances and illnesses that can affect this exposed organ in the most surprising ways, and about which there is little that can be done.

The most unusual documented example of injury to the penis is that of a fifty-four-year-old man from San Francisco who, after having a drink at his friendly bar, went into the bathroom, sat on the toilet, then flicked his cigarette into the bowl. The toilet exploded and literally blew him off the seat. What he didn't realize was that several hours earlier a young man had been cleaning out the gas tank of his motorcycle, and had emptied the dirty gasoline into the same toilet. But perils of the penis need not be so sudden or unlikely, and all men at various times in their lives will have to confront some of them.

* This chapter is dedicated to the late Dr. William Smart of San Rafael, California, who first coined this term.

Penile Amputation

It is amazing to doctors specializing in urology how infrequently the penis receives traumatic injury. Arms, legs, and fingers seem so easily injured, broken, or chopped off, but the penis seems to be protected most of the time. The main reported cases of total amputation of the penis have been in schizophrenic patients who intentionally severed their own organs. In two such cases, one in Boston and one in China, the tiny arteries that supply the penis with a rich flow of blood were reconnected under the microscope. But this is rare. Usually only a portion of the penis is cut because the penis slides away from the saw or the knife that is producing the injury. Whenever there is an incomplete amputation (whether of the finger or the penis), a few stitches through the skin to hold everything in place will allow partially severed organs to heal quite respectably. It is only in bizarre cases that a complete amputation is achieved and sophisticated replant surgery is necessary.

Bruises of the Penis

The penis appears to tolerate a great deal of trauma without injury. Just in thinking about the tremendous stress of intercourse, one can suddenly gain a great deal of respect for this rather durable structure. But sometimes things can go a little too far, and the penis does suffer some fairly painful bruises from overstrenuous activity. I recently saw a young man who had had an extraordinarily violent episode of intercourse a week earlier. He noted subsequently a large black and blue mark on the left side of his penis near the tip. In addition, there was a very hard, cordlike structure that could be felt all along the top of the penis. He was having normal erections since the episode, but was very worried about this cord, which ran all the way from the tip of the penis into his body. He was scared that he might have some sort of strange venereal disease, and was filled with guilt.

In fact, all that he had was a thrombosed dorsal penile vein. From extremely athletic intercourse, the penis can indeed be bruised, and the most typical reaction is that one of the major veins that brings blood back from the tip along the top of the penis becomes clotted and hard. Luckily there are so many extra veins that drain the blood from the penis that this traumatic thrombosis produces no problem except for a great deal of worry. It can be a little painful until it goes away, which may require as long as six to twelve weeks. This pain can be very scary unless one understands that it is the pain that any inflamed structure has to undergo while it is healing. It won't happen often, but when it does, men shouldn't worry that their penis is "broken." It is a resilient organ, and it will heal.

Twisted Penis (Peyronie's Disease)

A patient I treated recently first noted a small, hardened plaque underneath the skin of his penis in 1973. Over the next six months his penis began to curve in the direction of that plaque whenever he got an erection, and eventually his erections became painful. Then he developed plaques in other areas of the penis, and his erections began to bend and twist in a variety of directions. It almost began to look like a kudu horn whenever he got erect, and it became difficult for him to engage in intercourse. He was developing Peyronie's disease.

This disease can occur in any man from the ages of twenty to eighty, though it is most common between the ages of forty and fifty-five. It doesn't seem to be caused by any known infection, and indeed it is a medical mystery. All sorts of remedies bordering on witchcraft have been tried, usually with claims of dramatic success. However, none of these remedies has any scientific validity, and the reason they sometimes seem to work is that fortunately Peyronie's disease often goes away as quickly as it came. For some mysterious reason the hardened plaque begins to dissolve, the penis straightens out, and intercourse is possible once again. In other words, the cure rate of all the various witchcraftlike remedies is no greater than the cure rate in patients who are left completely untreated.

When this patient's penis first began to twist, he was given a drug called Potaba, the dosage consisting of twenty-four huge tablets a day. When that did no good, he was treated with large doses of vitamin E. Later he was placed on potassium pills, which caused stomach irritation and ulcers. His penis was then injected with steroids, which also did no good, and finally he was subjected to radiation therapy, which created a radiation burn on the surface but did nothing to cure the twisting. Six years later, after all this treatment had failed, he became completely impotent.

But Peyronie's disease does not always progress. It frequently improves spontaneously. Most patients whose Peyronie's disease ends happily begin to note improvement within a year. If several years have gone by and the condition continues to worsen, the outlook is poor. However, many men can have good erections despite a slight twist of the penis and can have excellent intercourse. So not everyone with Peyronie's disease needs an operation. Many men just learn to live with (and indeed enjoy) the new twist that they suddenly find themselves with.

I recently received an inquiry from a patient outside the United States who was thirty-four years old and terribly concerned about his Peyronie's disease. He reported that his doctor told him the only treatment would be radiation. When I talked to him personally, he confided that he was really having little difficulty with either erection or intercourse, but was mostly worried that if the angle of the erection became too acute, eventually he would not be able to have sex. This is the condition that most men with Peyronie's disease find themselves in, and it would be unfortunate for them to undergo unnecessary radiation, twenty-four pills a day, or, worst of all, unnecessary surgery. Pills and radiation don't work, and surgery is required only when the angle of the bend becomes so distorted that it makes intercourse impossible.

But frequently Peyronie's disease cures itself. A seventy-year-old man walked into my office a year ago. He was a nice, robust gentleman who had noticed a hardened lump on the upper portion of his penis that was beginning to cause it to bend upward at a severe angle when he got erect. Also, his erection was softer than it had been many years before, but it was still sufficient for penetration and intercourse. It would have been a mistake to treat this gentleman. He was having no difficulty with intercourse, but was understandably concerned and worried. He was treated with no medication and no surgery, but simply the assurance that something surgically could be done for him if the condition worsened. When I saw him a year later, the Peyronie's disease had gotten better without any treatment whatsoever, and there was no longer a lump or a twist to his erections.

Priapism—The Erection that Will Not Go Down

Priapism is a rare but absolutely horrifying condition wherein a man one day develops a very painful erection unaccompanied by any sexual excitation or desire. Occasionally priapism is caused by a blood disease like sickle cell anemia or leukemia, or it may result after very prolonged sexual stimulation, but in the vast majority of cases doctors have no idea why it develops.

Priapism results from the corporal bodies of the penis filling with blood under tremendous pressure, but without any of the drainage that normally occurs during an erection. The penis just keeps filling with blood and becomes super-engorged. If it is not treated promptly, the corporal bodies of the penis become a pool of noncirculating blood that over a period of a month will scar and cause complete obliteration of the normal spongy internal architecture. The patient becomes irrevocably impotent because there is no longer any normal channel left within his penis to fill with blood when he has sexual desire.

In a normal erection the two major corporal bodies of the penis and the corpus spongiosum surrounding the urinary tube are filled with blood. In priapism it is only the corporal bodies that fill with blood, and the spongy tissue surrounding the urinary tube is completely soft. From this knowledge has evolved a very simple emergency operation that can promptly cure the priapism. A small incision is made in the base of the penis, and a half-inch windowlike connection is made between the corporal bodies and the spongiosum. An enormous amount of blood is then released from this otherwise engorged penis through the window into the spongiosum. The erection immediately goes down, and when the patient awakes from anesthesia he has complete relief from his pain.

Patients operated on promptly will have their future potency preserved. Once priapism occurs, it is important not to dilly-dally. A painful erection unassociated with any sexual desire requires emergency surgery.

Lumps and Bumps and Rashes

Many lumps, bumps, and scaly, itchy growths that attack the penis are not in any sense venereal. Herpes of the penis and genital warts are in a sense venereal diseases even though the virus causing them might have originally arrived ten years earlier. It is difficult to think of herpes or warts as a venereal disease in the same sense as gonorrhea, where three days after beginning a new affair one suddenly has an infection and knows where it came from. Nonetheless, herpes and warts are venereal. Even with this broadened definition, however, most of the bumps and itchy, scaly skin problems that affect the penis are not truly venereal because they are not transmitted by intercourse.

A typical example of an itchy lesion that attacks many men at one time or another in their lives and is not venereal is *lichen planus*. It is very common. One day a man notices a small, ringwormlike, scaly, itchy area on the tip or even the shaft of his penis or scrotum. It develops a silvery, flaky appearance, and he really wonders where he picked this awful thing up. It itches terribly. Most men who get this come into the office with a tremendous amount of worry, anxiety, and confusion. It does not go away quickly, and it certainly will not respond to any antibiotic that a well-meaning doctor who isn't familiar with it may prescribe. Several weeks later the man begins to develop a similar type of itchy, scaly rash on his wrists and inside his mouth. A good dermatologist can diagnose this quickly. If untreated, it will go away in about eight to ten weeks, but steroid cream applied topically can hasten its resolution and relieve the itching. It is not venereal and it does not spread from one person to another.

Another itchy, scaly affliction of the penis is pityriasis rosea. Again, it is not venereal. The diagnosis is often missed by doctors because it can be confused with lichen planus, ringworm, scabies, or lice. Since pityriasis rosea affects other areas of the body as well, the man who has it may think it is some sort of disastrous infection spreading throughout his body. Doctors don't know what causes it, but they do know that it is not an infection, and it is not venereal. Furthermore, they know that with or without treatment it will go away by itself within four to eight weeks.

Making the proper diagnosis is very reassuring. The key to the diagnosis is remembering that about two weeks earlier there should have been a single, ringwormlike skin lesion on the arm or other part of the body, now almost forgotten and certainly unrecognized because it lasted only a few days and wasn't of enough consequence to remember. Two weeks after this so-called herald sign has been forgotten massive scaling and itching around the penis and other parts of the body suddenly develop. Recollection of the herald lesion establishes the correct diagnosis of pityriasis rosea, and allows the victim to relax and to wait for it to go away without any treatment.

Fungal infections, such as yeast and ringworm, are very common in the penis area. These are not truly venereal, but they can spread from one sexual partner to another. We all know how often women speak of the yeast infections that the gynecologists diagnose. These infections are minor but irritating. They are most likely to occur in women who are using birth control pills or who have diabetes or some other predisposing cause. They are not likely to attack her male partner unless he is uncircumcised. In an uncircumcised man the yeast find a very friendly environment in the area under the foreskin, but in circumcised men the yeast have a very difficult time finding a warm, wet foothold.

An entirely different kind of yeast infection is ringworm, or tinea cruris. This fungus infection is common in the groin area, a little bit removed from the scrotum and penis. Both the ringworm-type fungus and the yeast can produce similar itchy skin attacks. It is sometimes difficult for a doctor to make a clear differential diagnosis between ringworm and yeast. In the past that was important in deciding what treatment to use. The most effective agents for ringworm would not work on yeast infections, and the most common agents against yeast would not work on ringworm. But now there are creams, such as Lotrimin, Mica Tin, and Halotex, that are very effective against both yeast and ringworm. Thus, if the doctor makes a misdiagnosis of a yeast when it is really ringworm, it doesn't matter. Neither yeast nor ringworm can produce any permanent harm or damage to the genitals, but they can be extremely aggravating and itchy, and they are very common.

Molluscum Contagiosum

Molluscum contagiosum is a viral, wartlike skin disease most commonly found in children along the trunk and on the arms or legs. When it occurs in adults, it is found primarily in the genital area. In children it just passes from one child to another and is not venereal, but in adults it is transmitted sexually via the genitals. It infects only the most outer layer of skin. It takes about six weeks for these pearl-shaped bumps to erupt. They are painless, but they certainly look very worrisome.

In the past the standard treatment was to cut into them and dig them out of their base. The cheesy internal material would be scraped out of the inside and then they would heal over. Without such treatment these lesions stay for as long as a year. Untreated, they will eventually go away on their own, but imagine the aggravation and worry. Now there is a very simple remedy that bypasses surgery. A single drop of Spanish Fly—that is, a 0.7 percent cantharidin solution—will cause the lesions to dry up and completely disappear in just a few weeks. Many people have an old-fashioned notion that Spanish Fly is an aphrodisiac of some kind that creates an intense sexual appetite. In actuality, it is an extreme drying agent that, when given in too large a dose, can cause complete drying of the mucous membranes. Just a single drop on one of these warts will make it dry up and disappear without the need of surgery.

Warts

Warts on the penis are extremely common. They are as common as warts on the vagina. If they are located just inside the meatus (i.e., the opening that we urinate through) they are called venereal warts. If they are located on the outside of the penis they are called condyloma. There may be just one or two of these little bumps on the penis, or there may be hundreds. They can range from a minor irritation to a major disfigurement.

Fortunately, there are simple drugs (such as podophyllin, Cantharone, or 5-fluorouracil cream) that, when dabbed onto these warts, make them gradually disappear. In an occasional case of huge warts (called giant condyloma accuminatum) surgery may be necessary. Husband and wife may give these lesions to each other. Typically they are very minor and only a source of irritation and aggravation.

Herpes (Blebs)

Another, more frequent source of irritation to the penis is the now famous *herpes progenitalis*. Herpes is rapidly becoming one of the most common venereal diseases in our society. It is caused by a virus very similar to the one that causes cold sores on the mouth, and, like cold sores, it will not respond to any known antibiotic or any other treatment. Most venereal diseases respond to antibiotics, but herpes is virtually uncontrollable, and is thus a source of frantic concern to many people.

Herpes is not really dangerous or life threatening. It is usually localized to a few specific areas in the penis, and it usually goes away without treatment, only to come back at a later date, once again in the same spot. But it is so prevalent—20 percent of all sexually active males come in contact with it—so uncomfortable, and so worrisome that it is commanding a tremendous amount of national attention. (In fact, a new organization has been formed whose sole purpose is to disseminate information about herpes.) Patients have been treated with every type of therapy imaginable, but none of the readily available therapies is thought to be of any use, despite their widespread popularity. In most cases, herpes goes away no faster with all of the creams and ointments than it would if it were not treated at all.

Herpes is usually just an annoyance, but it can have some dangerous complications. The herpes virus may very well be one of the inciting agents that causes cancer of the cervix (the outlet of the female's womb). The wife of a man who has herpes probably has a greater chance of developing cancer of the cervix than a woman whose husband is free of the disease. If a woman has an active herpes eruption at the time that she is about to deliver her baby, it can cause severe damage to the baby as it passes through the birth canal, and the baby can develop a terrible case of herpes involving the eyes.

A minimum of five hundred thousand people develop herpes every year. Fortunately, the immune system in most people is strong enough to prevent herpes from gaining a foothold. But once it does, it never leaves. Never. Even though that first little herpes bleb on the penis disappears over the following seven to fourteen days, that doesn't mean it's gone. It simply remains dormant within the tiny nerve endings underneath the skin of the penis, until some day (a month or a year later) when the body's resistance is down, it will blossom forth again.

Herpes is no different from the common cold sore that many people get from time to time on their lips whenever their resistance is low. These cold sores used to be called herpes type I, while herpes cold sores on the penis, vagina, and cervix were called herpes type II. Herpes lesions above the waist were caused by a virus slightly different from the one that caused cold sores below the waist. But lately with the change in sexual habits and mores, virologists are noting that it is now common to find herpes type I on the penis and herpes type II (which was formely restricted to the genitals) in the mouth. Thus, the distinction between type I and type II is no longer valid.

The herpes virus often attacks during times of stress and tension as well as times of physical debilitation. When it does, a small, itchy swelling erupts somewhere around the surface of the penis, either at the tip or on the shaft, which eventually develops into a little bleb, and finally into tiny itching blisters that become very painful. It is when these blisters are wet, much like chicken pox in small children, that they are contagious. They do not disseminate throughout the body, but rather specifically reside in the region where they first appear.

Up until now no treatment has been satisfactory, though remarkable effects have been claimed for photoinactivation, Stoxyl, and even ether. For instance, some doctors claim that these remedies cause the lesions to go away faster and make them less likely to come back. But controlled studies have thus far not proved that the patients receiving any of these treatments have any faster remission of their disease than patients that receive no treatment at all.

Another new treatment that holds some promise is now being tried at the University of Pennsylvania in Philadelphia, but over the years there have been so many such treatments that it is easy to be skeptical. This treatment comes from well-respected biochemical virologists, though, and doctors will have to watch carefully to see whether it is any different from the many disappointments that herpes sufferers have experienced over the past twenty years.

Scabies and Crabs

Scabies and crabs are not really serious venereal diseases, in that they don't produce any permanent harm to the genitals, but they itch terribly, and can be incredibly aggravating and irritating. They are caused by tiny animals, parasites, that infest the skin of the genitals, and they are transmitted from one person to another by sexual contact.

Scabies is caused by the itch mite. The pregnant female mite burrows into the skin and deposits its eggs and feces. The baby mites then hatch in a little burrow under the skin, and move up to the surface where they develop into adult mites. Whenever there is close personal contact, such as with sexual intercourse, the female mites will travel from one individual to another, and the infection can start. The hallmark symptom of scabies is itching, which can become so intense at night that some of the skin of the penis is often actually torn off by the resultant scratching. The itch is caused by allergic sensitivity to the mite and its eggs, as well as its feces. The first time scabies are contracted, it takes several weeks for the itching to begin. But in future attacks, the itching starts almost immediately after sex. This is because the victim is already allergically sensitized to the scabies mite. The minute it begins to burrow and deposit its eggs and feces, the itching commences.

Fortunately, nowadays scabies can be easily treated with a lotion, or a shampoo, called Kwell (gamma benzene hexachloride). After a hot, clean bath, this Kwell lotion is applied to the entire body below the neck. The next day another hot bath is taken and new, freshly laundered clothing worn. Sometimes this regimen has to be repeated several times, but eventually the scabies will completely go away and the itching will be relieved. Kwell is very specific for killing these miserably aggravating parasites.

Crabs is very similar to scabies, but it is caused by a different parasite, called the crab louse. The crab louse specifically latches onto the hair and the skin of the pubic area. The female louse lays its eggs with a very hard covering so that they are attached firmly to the base of a single hair. The eggs hatch and the larvae develop into mature adults over the next two weeks. The adult louse is a sluggish, squat, crab-shaped creature that grabs onto two hairs with its four hind legs, one on each side of its body, by anchoring its mouth to the skin of the genitals. Most patients with these pubic lice are also infected with several other sexually transmitted venereal diseases. The lice are just part of the whole picture.

Crabs also causes itching and irritation but it is not nearly so severe as that caused by scabies. Sometimes the crabs just reside in the genitals asymptomatically, without producing any discomfort. The crab louse is actually visible to the naked eye. It can be a bit creepy to think of these little creatures crawling all over the crotch area. Once again, treatment with Kwell lotion should rid the victim of this awful nuisance.

Syphilis

Although we are experiencing an epidemic increase in venereal disease, syphilis, though one of the classic venereal diseases, is not really a part of this epidemic. Indeed, the total number of cases of syphilis per year has been declining steadily since 1963. Syphilis does remain a serious health problem among homosexuals, however. One-half of all cases of syphilis seen in New York City, and about 35 percent of all cases in the United States, occur in homosexuals. Otherwise, syphilis—unlike all other venereal diseases—is on the decline.

Syphilis used to be the most feared and dreaded disease in all of Europe. The French called it the English pox, figuring that it was brought over from England, and the English called it the French pox, deciding exactly the opposite. The disease took on many disguises and was often difficult to diagnose until twenty-five years after it was contracted, when it had already caused devastating disability from heart and brain damage. In fact, earlier in this century medical school professors always taught their students to consider syphilis in the diagnosis of any confusing illness. It was called the "great imitator," and it could rear its ugly head in almost any shape or form, frequently going undiagnosed. But today syphilis is regarded somewhat casually because its occurrence is declining so dramatically in the face of other venereal diseases.

Syphilis is relatively simple to treat. Any dose of penicillin or tetracycline will wipe it out completely. Actually, antibiotics such as penicillin and tetracycline are being handed out so indiscriminately by doctors around the country that if a person is carrying an undiagnosed case of syphilis, it would most probably at some time or other receive a dose of antibiotics that would eradicate it before it had a chance to do its later damage.

But despite its declining importance as a disease, syphilis remains one of the most fascinating and confusing perils of the penis ever known. It starts out as a small, painless, nickel-sized, button-shaped sore, usually on the tip of the penis and sometimes on the shaft, which develops between one week and three months following sex with a person who has syphilis or carries syphilis. This sore has a clearly delineated border and is remarkably pain free. The patient has no symptoms or other signs of illness. But this innocent little skin lesion on the penis is the beginning of a long and potentially frightening lifespan of the syphilis bacteria, which in twenty years may result in complete disability or death. The sore heals quickly without even leaving a scar. So ends the innocuous first stage of syphilis.

The second stage of syphilis begins several months later. Skin rashes develop all over the body which also are painless, unassuming, and not associated with any generalized fever, illness, or discomfort. Once again before a person even has a chance to consider the diagnosis, these rashes heal spontaneously without even leaving a scar or any sign that they were ever there. There is no characteristic appearance; they can look like almost anything. The diagnosis of this so-called secondary stage of syphilis is almost impossible unless the doctor and the patient are suspicious enough to order specific blood tests.

Following the disappearance of the skin lesions representing the second stage of syphilis, the patient remains asymptomatic, with no sign of any disease for several decades. After about twenty years have passed, one-third of these patients develop what is called the third stage of syphilis, or tertiary syphilis. For the previous twenty years the syphilis bacteria (called spirochetes) have been incubating in the central nervous system, the spinal cord, the brain, the heart, and the major blood vessels. For these twenty years, completely unknown to the victim, these little spiral-shaped, coiled bacteria have been slowly eating away at his tissues. In the third stage of syphilis, the victim finally evidences severe damage to the spinal cord, making it impossible to have proper sensation in the body; to the brain, causing mental disturbance; to the heart, causing leakage of the major valves; and to the major blood vessels, causing the deterioration of the wall of the aorta. Sometimes there can be damage to the liver, bones, spleen, and even the eyes, but these are less common than the brain, the heart, and the blood vessels.

Fortunately, if at any time during this entire asymptomatic twenty-year wait the patient is given a course of antibiotics, such as penicillin or tetracycline, all of these insidious little spirochetes that would otherwise eat out his insides are killed, and the final stage of syphilis will not develop.

The peculiar little coiled organism that causes this terrifying disease cannot live long outside of the human body, and certainly could not be transferred easily from a toilet seat because it is so delicate. It is not as hardy as other bacteria, and it is remarkable that such a weakling of an organism can unleash such deadly misery.

Gonorrhea

Gonorrhea is a terribly painful, miserable disease, and, unlike syphilis, it is still very common. About two million men (one in every hundred Americans) contract gonorrhea every year. Although this disabling venereal disease has usually been easily treated with penicillin, many Vietnam veterans brought home new varieties of gonorrhea that are resistant to penicillin. In fact, 2.5 percent of the enlisted men who returned from Vietnam had strains of gonorrhea, many of which had never before been seen in the United States.

Gonorrhea typically produces a copious, pussy, painful discharge from the tip of the penis within days of sexual contact. There is severe burning on urination, and the pain is intense. But not all men have these frank symptoms. Five percent of the men with this disease are actually asymptomatic carriers, transferring it to their partners without even knowing about it.

Gonorrhea can be devastating to the male genitals. As the infection heals, it can create scarring of the urethra (the tube of the penis through which the urine flows), and this can make urinating extremely difficult, often causing other infections and requiring extensive surgery. Gonorrhea can also cause blockage of the sperm-carrying ducts, particularly the delicate epididymis that conveys sperm from the testicle into the vas deferens (see page 6).   Indeed, in some communities in Africa, where gonorrhea has absolutely run rampant due to inadequate antibiotic control, as many as 30 percent of the men are completely sterile from obstruction of the sperm ducts caused by gonorrhea. Gonorrhea can cause painful swelling of the vas deferens, epididymis, and testicles. Occasionally it can even spread via the bloodstream to bones and joints in far removed areas of the body.

Gonorrhea can also be found in the rectum and in the throat. It can be transferred to any of these areas via sexual contact. Unlike syphilis, gonorrhea has been steadily increasing in this country over the years.

It is very easy for a doctor to make the diagnosis of gonorrhea by simply looking at a stained specimen of your penile discharge under a microscope, where the dot-shaped, paired bacteria that cause gonorrhea can be easily seen. These bacteria can also be cultured by routine techniques available in most laboratories.

Although gonorrhea and syphilis are considered the classic venereal diseases, gonorrhea is in no way similar to syphilis, except in that both diseases are transmitted by sexual activity and that both are highly contagious. Incidence of gonorrhea is increasing not only because of the widening variety of sexual experience that most young men now have, but also because condoms are now used much less frequently for birth control. Condoms not only prevented the sperm from getting out and causing pregnancy, but they also prevented the bacteria from getting in.

With about 10 percent of teenage girls getting pregnant, many married men and women having extramarital relationships, and most heterosexual men having had several sexual partners by the time they marry, as well as the appearance of gonorrhea in children as young as thirteen years of age in New York City, we can see how easy it is for these organisms to gain a firm foothold and continually increase their prevalence in our society.

Nonspecific Urethritis

By far the most common of all venereal diseases is nonspecific urethritis. This disease is similar to gonorrhea except that it is usually much milder. It is rarely painful, but it can still be insidiously destructive. For some reason or other, this nonspecific urethritis is much more common in white, affluent men than is the gonorrheal variety. In any event, cases of nonspecific urethritis outnumber gonorrheal urethritis by at least two to one.

Over the past ten years there has been a spectacular increase in the number of cases of nonspecific urethritis. All urologists across the country report that this is the most common cause of urethral drip and burning of the penis on urination. This nonspecific form of urethritis does not respond to penicillin at all. It may go away by itself, slowly. The proper treatment is not penicillin but rather tetracycline, an entirely different antibiotic. Men who are given penicillin injections for what is thought to be a mild form of gonorrhea frequently never get better because they do not in truth have gonorrhea. Rather they have the nonspecific form of urethritis that requires a different antibiotic. When a man comes into the doctor's office with a drip from his penis, the doctor takes a smear and looks at it under the microscope. He is looking for gonorrhea. If he doesn't find those little dot-shaped bacteria that come in pairs located inside the inflammatory cells of the discharge, then he concludes that this is not gonorrhea, but rather a nonspecific urethritis.

In the past, doctors were really in a complete cloud as to what kind of organism causes this infection. They didn't even know whether it was venereal or not, but now much of that mystery has been solved. Nonspecific urethritis is caused in at least 40 percent of all cases by an unusual organism called chlamydia. This is a bacterialike organism that cannot be cultured by most laboratories in the United States and cannot be seen routinely under the microscope. This mysterious organism had been eluding doctors for many years as they wondered how men could have urethral discharge and painful urination, indicating the probability of venereal disease, and yet have no detectable gonorrheal organisms. These patients usually responded to tetracycline, and yet doctors never had any idea why.

Chlamydia can only live and multiply inside living cells. In this respect it is a bacterium that behaves like a virus. If doctors attempt to culture it in a standard laboratory, it will not grow. Furthermore, if they try to see it under the microscope, they find that it can barely be seen even by the most experienced clinicians. There are only a few laboratories in the country that are truly capable of culturing, isolating, and identifying these mysterious organisms. Therefore, the diagnosis is simply made on clinical suspicion plus the failure to identify gonorrhea. Fortunately, almost all cases respond to the simple and common antibiotic tetracycline.

The fact that this much more prevalent type of venereal disease, nonspecific urethritis, seems to be so mild in its presenting symptoms is no reason to be nonchalant or relaxed about obtaining treatment. Though less painful than gonorrhea, it can have the same disastrous effect on the genitals, causing scarring of the urinary tube, sperm ducts, and epididymis. It is simply a slower, more insidious process than gonorrhea.

6

Impotence and the Mind

All men sometime in their lives are going to lose their erection, at least temporarily, in the course of making love. This is a common and normal event that every man at one time or another is going to endure. The danger is that this temporary loss of erection can cause such haunting fears of waning erectile powers, and declining sexuality, that the fear itself can escalate into a permanent psychological impotence. A single transient episode of failure can cause a man such tension and worry about his performance that he tends to focus all of his thinking on his erection. It is the fear of failure that ensures failure.

Changes in Male Sexuality with Age

As men get older, the thing they fear most is that they may become impotent. This fear is reinforced by the painful but inescapable realization that every year after the age of twenty the force of male sexuality slowly diminishes. Although men should be potent and enjoy a good sex life into old age, it is obvious that with each succeeding decade things just aren't quite as they were in earlier years. The speed with which they are sexually aroused, the rapidity of obtaining a firm erection, the ability to achieve an orgasm, the length of time necessary after an orgasm before they are able to get another erection, and even the force of the ejaculatory squirt at the time of orgasm diminish gradually as the years go by. Men in their late thirties or forties often wonder just how much more time is left. This fear, brought on by physical changes beyond their control, can so unnerve them that they may become so self-conscious that they are not able to get an erection at all. In most cases, impotence is all in the mind. The brain is the most important sex organ.

It is ironic how poorly Mother Nature seems to have organized the sexual responses of men and women at different ages. Men reach the height of their physical sexuality in their late teens, then gradually decline throughout the rest of their lives. On the other hand, women in our culture undergo a slow increase in their sexuality, which reaches maximum in their late thirties and early forties. By the time women reach their maximum sexuality, men are already in a state of decline. It is possible that this change in women is purely a cultural one and not physically inevitable in all societies. But the decline in male sexuality with age is a physical inevitability that is inescapable. If this decline is understood, a man can continue to have a great sex life into his eighties; but if it is not understood, intense frustration can result (at the same time that his mate's sexuality is increasing), and this can turn him off completely. This is probably the most common cause of impotence. Impotence is usually a psychosomatic disease, but its roots are frequently in normal physical deterioration that most men do not expect and cannot handle.

Male infants are capable of having firm erections from birth, although the cause of these prepubertal erections is poorly understood. At puberty, with the sudden release of testosterone from the testicles, boys develop a dramatic libido. Although there is a large variation from individual to individual in the time of sexual peak, clearly by age seventeen or eighteen, most boys have an intense adolescent sexual drive, resulting in erections at the

slightest provocation, relatively frequent masturbation, and sometimes a genuine difficulty in coping with these intense new hormonal urges. Both the original studies of Kinsey and the subsequent studies by Masters and Johnson have confirmed that male
physical sexuality is maximum at age seventeen or eighteen, with
a slow, steady decline thereafter.

In all men there is a refractory period immediately after
orgasm, during which time they are unable to get another erection. For men in their thirties, this refractory period can last from
several hours to half a day, but for boys in their teen years, it can
be as short as a few minutes. Erection in the teenager is an instantaneous response to any kind of psychic or physical stimulation,
and frequently the young man is embarrassed by the erection
showing through his pants at inappropriate times. Furthermore,
after orgasm the teenager's erection may be slow in going down,
whereas for men in their thirties or forties, the erection goes down
almost instantaneously following orgasm.

For young men the orgasm is extremely intense, with a very
forceful spurt, which can propel the ejaculate as far as a foot or
two. In older men the ejaculate comes out less forcefully, and in
very old men there is often just a little seepage of fluid to represent the ejaculation. In young men, one to three seconds before
ejaculation there is a sense of an ejaculatory inevitability—the
highly pleasurable feeling derived from contraction of the seminal
vesicles and the vas deferens squirting sperm and fluid into the
bulb at the base of the penis. The actual ejaculation follows this
sensation and a very powerful compression of the muscles around
the base of the penis then squirts out the semen. Older men do
not experience these two distinct phases of orgasm as crisply as
do young men.

It is usually when a man passes the age of forty that he
notices a distinct difference in the quality of his sexuality. After
the age of fifty most men cannot redevelop an erection for half a
day to a full day after their last ejaculation, and much longer and
more intense stimulation is necessary to achieve an erection and
ejaculation. During early love play, a man in his fifties usually no

longer erects the second he touches his partner's body. He may require a considerable amount of stimulation and fondling before his erection is actually firm enough for penetrating the vagina. Although the man in his teens and twenties will often desire sex every night or every other night if he has a partner available, the man in his fifties frequently can become involved in his work and go for weeks without an erection or even a thought of sex.

In a sense, then, there is a male menopause, which in many respects can be more devastating than the female menopause. It is not caused by a decline in hormone production from the testicles, because the male continues to produce his sex hormones in essentially normal amounts throughout life, despite going through a very clear-cut change in sexuality as he gets older.

Although the female hormones suddenly cease to be produced when a woman goes through menopause, the female menopause is not associated with any significant decline in sexuality. The male menopause can be devastating because it truly reflects a declining sexuality to which the man must adjust mentally. But most men should be able to enjoy sexual intercourse throughout life, despite these changes. No longer having the intense and uncontrollable need for a quick orgasm, and being perhaps more mature in his relationships, he may be able to enjoy love play and sexuality even more. If he is insecure and fears that his declining sexual performance is making him less of a man, this fear in itself will usually cause him to be impotent. If he can learn to understand these changes without fear and insecurity, his sexual pleasure may, if anything, improve rather than decline with age.

Changes in Female Sexuality with Age

Our information about female sexuality is scientifically less reliable than our information about males, because so much of it may be culturally induced and subject to change as our culture changes. Girls in their teen years tend to have a somewhat less intense awakening of sexuality than boys. For example, 95 percent of boys masturbate in their teen years, whereas only 30 to 40 percent of teenage girls report any sort of masturbatory experience. The early experiences that young girls have with sex are usually disappointing, because they rarely reach orgasm. Although early in her marital years a young woman's frequency of intercourse is at its peak (two to five times per week), it is primarily motivated by the intense sex drive of her young husband. He wants to have sex frequently, obtains his erection instantly, reaches orgasm soon after vaginal penetration, and frequently simply leaves his young wife unsatisfied.

Ironically, women in our culture tend to reach their peak sexuality in their early forties, just when the man's sexuality is declining. In fact, from a purely physiological point of view, the woman's sex drive, her libido, should *increase* rather than decrease when she undergoes menopause because the male hormone that her adrenal gland produces (which is responsible for her sexual drive) is no longer being counteracted by her female hormones, estrogen and progesterone. It is only the fear that age may be decreasing her physical attractiveness that may interfere with a woman's sexuality as she gets older. Her actual desire for sex does not decline.

A woman in her late thirties or early forties is capable of multiple and frequent orgasms with no refractory period. Even in old age women are able to have multiple orgasms during intercourse, as opposed to elderly men who simply have one orgasm, which may take them a long time to achieve, and after which they are certainly unable to achieve another erection until the next day at the earliest.

As a couple gets older, the wife's increasing intensity of sexual interest may combine with the husband's somewhat decreased speed in obtaining erection to cause the husband to feel tremendous pressure to perform, and this can create a great fear of failure. Furthermore, the husband's need for greater stimulation in order to obtain an erection can be interpreted by his wife to mean that he is less aroused by her than he once was and finds her less adequate as a sexual partner. Both the man and the woman in the relationship are undergoing biological changes that neither of them understands and that may be interpreted by them in such a way as to put great pressure on the relationship—pressure so great and anxiety so overwhelming that the man often becomes unable to perform at all.

How to Tell Whether Impotence Is Psychological or Organic

There are some cases of impotence caused purely by physical factors, and psychological insight will not give a man with such problems back his erections. Disease processes such as blockage of blood flow, neurologic disorders, and diabetes can cause organic impotence. Chronic alcoholism, general illness, and even some medications may contribute to organic impotence or aggravate psychologically induced impotence. For men with true organic impotence the only hope is surgery (see Chapter 7). But for the majority of men with impotence, surgery is unnecessary because the impotence is all mental.

How do we know when impotence is purely psychological? There is a simple test that can be performed at any time in a man's life when he discovers that he can't obtain an erection. This test is frequently therapeutic as well. Just the realization that his penis is all right can give a man enough reassurance that his erections will return quickly. (This test was discussed in greater detail in Chapter 2, and is repeated here because of its importance to those worried about impotence.)

All men normally have about five firm erections every night while they are sleeping, which they usually don't know about. Every ninety minutes during the night, our sleep goes through a phase called rapid eye movement sleep (REM sleep), during which men get a good, stiff erection that lasts usually for about half an hour. This phenomenon occurs regularly and repeatably every night no matter how nervous or tense they might be, and no matter what difficulties they might be having in obtaining an erection while awake. If they happen to wake up during an REM sleep period, they will have a firm erection. Men who are biologically unable to obtain an erection because of some disease process, such as a blockage of blood flow, neurologic disorder, or diabetes, do not have erections at night while they are sleeping. But men who are psychologically impotent will have good, firm erections every night as they sleep.

There is an easy way for a man to use these nightly erections to find out whether his impotence is psychological or organic. All he need do is take a roll of postage stamps and wrap it in a single thickness around the shaft of the penis, tearing off the excess stamps before taping the two ends around the penis firmly, though not too tight. Then he simply goes to sleep. When a nighttime erection occurs, the increased diameter of the penis should break the stamps along the line of one of the perforations. If a man is not having nightly erections, or if his erections are very weak, then when he wakes in the morning, he will find the stamps still rolled around his penis, undisturbed.

This process can be repeated every night for as long as a month to determine just how regular and how frequent a phenomenon it is. If a man regularly finds the stamps broken along the perforations in the morning, he can feel fairly confident that he has a normal capability for having erections, and is simply failing under the stressful circumstances of attempting to make love.

I recently had a seventy-two-year-old patient who was very concerned because he just didn't seem to be able to get erections and have intercourse anymore. He had been placed on hormone supplements by some doctors, told to relax by others, and had even been offered surgery by still others. But no one had ever checked to see whether or not he had nocturnal erections. I told him about the stamp test and made arrangements for him to come back to the office for further counseling in a month. When he walked into the office one month later he had a big smile on his face and told me he really didn't think it was necessary to come back anymore, but just wanted to let me know how everything worked out. His stamp test had been positive for twenty-nine days in a row. He was so elated and had such a boost in his confidence after discovering that he could have normal erections that he was able to have sex regularly and with no difficulty. Not all cases of psychological impotence clear up quite this quickly, easily, or dramatically, but this case does point out what an important first step the impotent man takes by finding out for sure that his penis is all right, and that his problem is truly in his head.

Last year I saw a typical example of a patient who was confused and unable to solve his problem because it was simply not clear either to him or his previous doctors whether his problem was psychological or organic. He was a forty-three-year-old man with diabetes. It is well known that about 50 percent of such long-term diabetic men have organic impotence. The little blood vessels that supply blood to the main chambers of the penis become scarred by the diabetic process. Even some of the nerves that regulate erection can be affected by the disease. Yet the man's history sounded as though he also had some sexual inhibitions and psychological problems that could have caused the impotence.

Rather than speculate about whether difficulties he was having with his sexual partner or his anxiety about intercourse was causing his impotence, or whether it was simply his diabetes, I told him to perform the stamp test on himself every night for the next month. When he came back to see me a month later, he reported that the stamp test had been positive every night and that he now knew he could have good erections. His problem was not organic impotence caused by diabetes. Indeed, someday he may become organically impotent because he is a diabetic, and he may then need an operation, but at least for the present the stamp test was able to let him know that his penis was still all right. If he could learn to deal with his anxiety about sex, he would be able to enjoy it once again and have no difficulty obtaining erections.

The Psychology of Erection

When a man wants to lift his arm up, he simply sends directions from his brain to his arm and his arm lifts up. When he wants to swallow, his brain simply gives directions to the muscles of his throat, and he swallows. When he wishes to urinate, his brain gives directions to his bladder, and he urinates. These actions are under his voluntary control. However, he has no voluntary control over such actions as his heartbeat, sweating, or even the contraction of the pupils of his eyes when he enters a dark room.

In a similar manner, a man has no voluntary control over his erections. It is impossible to will an erection. An erection does not occur simply because a man's brain gives a direction to his penis that he would like to have an erection. He has no conscious control over it. However, when he feels sexually aroused by the sight of his partner, or because of sensuous fondling of his penis, an erection occurs all on its own, involuntarily. If he tries to will an erection, or demand that his penis get ready for intercourse, it simply will not happen. When a man tries to insert his voluntary control into the process because he is so worried that it will not take place properly otherwise, he is interfering with the normal sequence of events that is psychologically mediated by areas of the brain that are not under his conscious direction.

A man can inhibit an erection easily enough, but it requires a certain degree of abandonment and willingness to let whatever may happen happen, in order for his penis to respond in the natural fashion to erotic sensation by becoming erect. It is as hopeless for him to try to make his penis become erect by thinking about it as it is for an insomniac to fall sleep by thinking about it.

This concept is one of the foundations of a whole new revolution in helping people with sexual difficulties. It is one of the principal pillars of sex therapy introduced by Masters and Johnson in the late sixties, and practiced now by sex therapists all around the country. The prevalent viewpoint before the era of Masters and Johnson was that anyone with psychological impotence had a deep-seated conflict far back in his brain and deeply rooted in his relationship with his partner. All of those deep psychological conflicts would have to be solved by extensive psychotherapy so as to correct the individual's underlying psychiatric disturbance. Once that had been achieved, then supposedly his erections would come back naturally, and he would again be able to have effective sexual relations.

The new sex therapists don't dispute that the psychological problems leading to impotence may be deeply rooted in a man's unconscious, but they question whether he has to dig all that up to solve the immediate problem of impotence. The new sex therapists take the pragmatic point of view that simple problems like fear of failure or the patient thinking too much about whether or not he can get an erection can be corrected fairly easily and promptly with simple behavioral techniques, without the need for expensive, drawn-out psychiatric treatment. The symptoms of sexual dysfunction and impotence may very well be part of larger issues within the person's life, gigantic intrapsychic conflicts, or marital conflicts that interfere with sexuality. But in most instances, there has been dramatic success in alleviating impotence with counseling techniques, which just remove the fear of failure.

Remedies for Psychological Impotence

There are several specific types of thinking patterns that cause most cases of impotence, and which can be corrected. They all tend to involve the "fear of failure" and anxiety about the ability to perform sexually. Here are some of those difficulties and what simple steps may be taken to alleviate them.

In the first place, many couples quite seriously don't know how to provide sensitive, sexual stimulation to their partners. They simply do not know how to make love. The young husband may not be aware of the foreplay, caressing, and fondling of the wife's genitals that may be necessary to begin her slow phase of vaginal swelling and lubrication, which is her equivalent of his getting an erection. The young husband may not understand this because his erection is almost instantaneous and his goal may be to penetrate her vagina immediately.

The wife may become unresponsive to such crude and ineffective lovemaking, and her lack of response can then turn the husband off to the point where he is not adequately stimulated. The older husband who has been accustomed for many years to having a rapid erection at the immediate touch of his wife may not realize that he needs more stimulation now to function, and his wife may not realize it either. Whereas in their youth he had to be willing to engage in an adequate amount of foreplay to heighten her sexual arousal, now he is dependent upon foreplay for *his* arousal as well. In this kind of poor lovemaking situation, the solution is simply for the couple to communicate, and to learn how to stimulate and explore each other.

Another misunderstanding in the technique of lovemaking is the erroneous notion in our culture that mutual and simultaneous orgasm is the ultimate goal of sexual intercourse. This is a difficult goal to reach, and its quest can lead to a lot of anxiety and, again, inadequate lovemaking. If the husband is always concentrating on holding back his orgasm because he knows his wife will take somewhat longer to reach her climax, and if she is striving intellectually as hard as she can to try to reach her orgasm hurriedly for fear that she might be too late, sex becomes difficult to enjoy. Again, the result of this anxiety may be impotence. There is simply a lot of misinformation about sex, and misinformation can frequently be the major cause of the man's failure to get an erection. If the man and the woman cannot discuss their desires openly, they each begin to have doubts about the other's feelings. Then the problem may become unsolvable unless a third party intervenes.

The most common cause of impotence is not poor sexual technique, but simply the fear of failure: a man's anxiety over whether his sexual performance will be adequate. If he feels that a proper sexual performance is being demanded by his partner, the fear that he will be rejected if he does not supply it makes it impossible for him to perform at all. Impotence is frequently caused by viewing sex as a performance.

The most effective method of removing anxiety is to prohibit intercourse temporarily. Patients with psychological impotence are told by their sex therapist that they must not have intercourse. They are instructed, together with their sexual partner, to do anything else they want to do to give each other erotic pleasure. They can fondle and kiss each other's genitals, and engage in any kind of gentle non-stress-oriented display of affection, but they are not allowed to have intercourse. Thus, from the very beginning the man is no longer on stage, and no longer has pressure placed upon him to get an erection. He can use his hands or his mouth or any other method of expressing affection to provide erotic pleasure for his partner, but he is not allowed to use his penis. Furthermore, his female partner is encouraged to do whatever she can to provide erotic pleasure for him, but without ever asking for vaginal penetration.

This period of prohibition of intercourse can last anywhere from two to six weeks. During that time the ability to have erections will usually return. There is then a great temptation for the man who finds that he can perform once again to violate this prohibition from intercourse. Sometimes this is all right, but frequently immediate return to anxiety about performance will once again cause failure. There has to be a period of restoration of confidence, with mutual-pleasure-providing sexual "tasks," before intercourse is finally allowed. The couples must engage in mutual nondemanding pleasuring experiences, where the goal of genital stimulation is not to produce an orgasm but simply to create a sense of nonorgasmic erotic pleasure.

At least half of the male population has experienced occasional transient episodes of impotence. It is perfectly normal for this harrowing event to occur from time to time in the lives of all men. The problem occurs when it creates such anxiety, worry, and insecurity over future performance that suddenly the man finds that what was simply a transient event is now persisting. The impotent man usually feels aroused sexually, but his penis simply doesn't cooperate. Sometimes even though the man is unable to get an erection he can still ejaculate. Sometimes he obtains his erection easily at first but then loses it at a specific time during the sexual act. Some men lose their erection just as they are about to enter the vagina, some men have only partial erections, and some only experience impotence with specific partners and not with others.

In all of these situations, it is the man's fear of sexual failure, the pressure of sexual demands, and the inability to let go of his consciousness about his own sexual feelings that cause the problem. The role of sex therapists in trying to cure impotence is to create a nondemanding sexual climate, where the man is not evaluating or watching his own performance but simply focuses his mind on the erotic sensations of pleasure derived by his mate's fondling. The man in his forties may resent being told that this is all psychological, because he "knows" that something in him is different physically than it used to be. Of course. Sexually he simply is not the same man he was twenty years ago. But the fact that he no longer can get an erection adequate for intercourse is not physical and is not related to age, but rather to the genuine fear and stress created by his awareness that his sexuality is diminished from earlier days.

Premature Ejaculation

Premature ejaculation is another common male sexual problem. There is a lot of controversy over what causes men to ejaculate prematurely, but it is one of the easiest sexual problems to cure with simple behavior modification, or, in simpler terms, conditioning. Let's explain what behavior modification is all about. You may have heard about the famous experiment with Pavlov's dog. Whenever Pavlov brought food to his dog, the dog would begin to salivate in anticipation of his meal. Pavlov then rang a bell every time he brought food to the dog. Eventually, the dog would salivate when Pavlov simply rang the bell even when there was no food. This is called conditioned response or, as any athlete will know, training. You can train people to play a piano, improve their tennis, and even delay ejaculation. Ejaculation can come under voluntary control once a man learns to observe his own sexual excitement sufficiently that just prior to the expected moment of ejaculatory inevitability he can concentrate on not letting go.

In some men premature ejaculation is so severe that the moment they get an erection they ejaculate immediately and it is all over. In other men a little bit of foreplay takes place, but for some reason just prior to entrance of the vagina they ejaculate, and again cannot consummate intercourse. In other patients vaginal penetration takes place, but excitement is so out of control that after merely a few pelvic thrusts the man has his orgasm, and his partner certainly is not satisfied. In the majority of men with this problem ejaculation takes place just prior to or immediately after entering the vagina.

No one really knows why men have premature ejaculation, though there is certainly an abundance of theories and ideas. Luckily none of these theories really matters, because treatment with behavior therapy is so successful. Masters and Johnson first described what they call the "squeeze" technique. The husband lies down on his back naked, and his wife, who is facing him straddled by her husband's legs, stimulates his penis until he begins to perceive that orgasm is soon going to be inevitable. At that point he must give her a signal and in response to the signal she stops stimulating the penis and instead squeezes it just below the tip with enough force to cause him to lose his erection. She doesn't do this with malice or with intent to hurt, but simply squeezes firmly enough that the erection will go down. Then when his fear that he is about to ejaculate is over she begins to stimulate him sexually again. Once again when he gives the signal that orgasm is imminent she squeezes the penis and again the erection goes down and he doesn't ejaculate. After a while the man is able to control ejaculation. Then they try intercourse. As soon as he feels that he is about to climax the wife withdraws his penis immediately and squeezes it until he loses erection. Masters and Johnson have reported that in just two weeks, 98 percent of men with premature ejaculation are cured with this approach.

It is amazing that this simple training procedure seems to work so well in curing premature ejaculation, whereas complex, long-term, expensive psychotherapy to alleviate the basic underlying anxieties that supposedly cause the problem has been ineffective. By using this simple behavioral approach a man is able to focus his attention upon the sensations that immediately precede orgasm, and this kind of "biofeedback" allows him to exercise voluntary control over it. This type of treatment is not very much different from the simple approach to bed-wetting described later in this book. Again, in that case the concept has evolved that whatever form of anxiety it may be that is causing the problem, long-term psychotherapy is not going to do as much good as short-term training.

It is interesting that the more one thinks about having an orgasm and trying to have an orgasm, the more difficult it may be. Sometimes wanting to have an orgasm can make one concentrate so much on it that he may have a great deal of difficulty. In some men the inhibition is so strong that they can't ejaculate while making love to their partner, and literally must leave the room and masturbate in order to obtain orgasm and relieve their sexual tension. The problem of retarded ejaculation is a difficult one and perhaps ultimately can only be solved by a close communication and interchange between the man and his partner. It is quite a different story from premature ejaculation, which is one of the simplest of all male sex problems to alleviate.

It should be clear by now, however, that although the penis is the most obvious of the male sex organs, the mind is certainly the most important one.

Size of the Penis

Of the many unwarranted fantasies and fears men have about their sexual adequacy, concern about the size of the penis is the most common. Young men often worry about whether their penis is long enough for them to be good lovers, and this worry can be a factor in psychologically induced impotence.

In most of the animal world the male's ability to reproduce depends on his ability to attract discriminating females toward him. The plumage of birds, the horns of some hoofed mammals, and the hornlike weapons of certain insects confer upon the males a quality of attractiveness to the female that is critical to survival. Thus there is a certain biological argument, beginning with Darwin, that females are attracted to the male with the most impressive assembly of parts. But physical attributes are not the sole factors by which choice of a mating partner is made, particularly not in so complex an animal as man. Recent studies on the black-tipped hanging fly have demonstrated that the female chooses her mate not on the basis of the attractiveness of his sexual accessories, but rather on the size of the prey that he provides for her during courtship. Indeed, the length of time and the enthusiasm with which she makes love with a male depend not on the quality of his sex organs, but rather on the size of his offering. In the same way it is a man's general qualities as an individual, not the size of his penis, that will make him attractive to a woman.

Several years ago my office received a call from a man in Rio de Janeiro who wanted to fly all the way to St. Louis to see me for an office visit. He was unwilling to state his problem over the phone, but he seemed so insistent that he was given an appointment. We had no idea why he wanted to see me and he refused to write or say anything over the phone about what his problem was. So he flew eight thousand miles to St. Louis from Rio de Janeiro, and I saw him in my office. When we were in the examining room, he quietly explained that his penis was "too small." He explained to me how important it was to be macho in Brazil, and how difficult his sex life had become because his penis was "so small."

Much to my surprise when I examined him, his penis was actually quite large, longer than six inches in a nonerect state. Yet he looked at it and said to me, "Isn't it disgraceful, it is so small?" I explained to him that there was nothing I could do to lengthen it. He seemed disappointed. Then he calmly put his pants back on, walked out the door, and flew back to Brazil. He had several operations performed in Brazil in an effort to lengthen his penis, none of which was ever satisfactory. Amazingly and luckily, he did not lose his potency from these futile operations, but this man will never be happy, always thinking that his genitalia are somehow not adequate.

Size is purely a matter of vanity. There is a great deal of variation in the size of penises and it is very difficult to define what is too small or, for that matter, what is too large. Size has nothing to do with sexual pleasure for either partner. Obesity, in fact, is more likely to interfere with sexual intercourse, by obscuring and hiding the penis under a roll of fat, than the actual size of the penis.

Urologists all over the country see patients who blame an inadequate sex life, a poor marriage, or even their impotence on the fact that their penis is too small. They frequently get calls from patients who want a "penile transplant," because they are hoping this will somehow lengthen their penis and improve their masculine attractiveness. Not only is this surgery unavailable, but if it were, it would not improve their attractiveness any more than the male black-tipped hanging fly's attractiveness would be improved by its having a longer proboscis.

7

Surgery for Impotence, or the Inflatable Erection

Inability to obtain an erection is one of the most disturbing events in a man's life. For the man whose failure to achieve erection is simply a temporary psychological problem, the impotence is simply a scary episode that makes him appreciate the marvelously complicated functioning of his penis. However, if his impotence is not such a psychological event, the frustration can be overwhelming.

Organically impotent men are usually able to ejaculate; they just cannot get an erection. For these patients there are now surgical procedures that can allow them to once again have good erections and normal intercourse. There are all kinds of internal silicone devices, some with hinges and some that are inflated by pumping a little bulb in the scrotum. These surgically implantable devices all work much like the penis bone that provides erections in other animals, such as bears, walruses, and dogs.

Early Surgical Efforts

Operations to correct impotence date back to the late 1800s, though only in the last five years has surgery been truly effective.

In 1889 the famous Dr. Brown-Sequard ground up dog's testicles and injected an extract of this preparation into himself through a hypodermic needle. He then stated that he regained his former strength, fatigued less easily, was able to work harder, noted an increase in his mental ability, and was even relieved of constipation. Of course, we now know that this extract could have had no such effect other than psychological, like a placebo. In the 1920s a Dr. Steinach performed vasectomies on bulls, rams, and senile rats, maintaining that these old animals became rejuvenated, sexually and otherwise, by vasectomy. This became known as the Steinach operation, written up widely in the *Journal of the American Medical Association* in 1912 and 1914. According to these early sex doctors, "The heart is invigorated, the pulse becomes regular, circulation improves, arterial tension is reduced to normal, headache and vertigo disappear, appetite is improved, metabolism is increased, calcareous deposits in arteries and joints are absorbed, musculature is strengthened, gait is made firm and upright, sleep is restored through decreased nocturnal micturition and clearness of thought and ability to undertake intellectual work is restored," by bilateral vasectomy. It was not until the 1940s that doctors realized that this operation as a method of restoring lost potency was absurd.

Another early effort to restore potency through surgery was attempted by Dr. Serge Voronoff of Paris in 1918. He announced that potency and youth could be restored to middle-aged men by implanting monkey testicles into the patient's scrotum. In the United States, Dr. Laspinasse, Professor of Urology at Northwestern University in Chicago, was at that time a leading proponent of his approach. First he attempted to have his impotent patients swallow an extract of monkey testicle, but finally in 1918 he recommended grafting slices of human testicle from a fresh cadaver. In 1922 Dr. Stanley at the San Quentin prison in California performed such procedures on over six hundred patients, seven of whom were women. However, Dr. Stanley did not use human cadaver testicles as did Professor Laspinasse of Northwestern University. Instead, he used the testicles of goats, rams, boars, and deer. Testicles of these animals were diced and then placed in a pressure syringe for injection just underneath the skin of the impotent patient. The results of this procedure were nothing short of miraculous. He reported marked improvement in vision, rheumatism, acne, diabetes, tuberculosis, senility, impotence, and sexual desire. Clearly in those early days the surgical treatment of impotence was pure witchcraft, even in the hands of otherwise respected physicians. Any success with these absurd methodologies would have to have been due to the placebo effect in patients whose only problems were psychological.

Another operation in the early 1900s, popularized at the University of Illinois by a well-known professor of surgical urology at that institution, Dr. Lydston, was to tie off one of the veins that drain blood from the penis. This was supposed to cause the impotent penis to fill with blood and become erect more easily. Though some scientific colleagues severely questioned his approach, the doctor defended himself with an emotional pontification rather than cold logic: "The patient wants relief, not a psychic diagnosis. Scientific reasoning and psychopathic diagnosis fall to the ground before the absolute of a flaccid penis in a physiological emergency." The doctor was serious when he said that.

The concept of blocking the veins of the penis makes little sense. A normal erection occurs because the two cavernous bodies of the penis fill with an enormous amount of blood that has a difficult time getting out. If the penis filled with blood because the veins that drained it closed during the moment of sexual desire, it would certainly be understandable why a surgeon would tie off the veins to block the drainage of blood. What the surgeons of the early 1900s did not realize, however, is that the major cause of erection is a tremendous increase in the flow of blood to the penis rather than a decreased return of blood out of it. In fact, if all that was required to induce an erection was to block the egress of blood from the penis, one could simply put a rubber band around it. However, that does not work either.

These witchcraftlike operations only worked in those men with purely psychological impotence who responded as to a placebo. None of the men with truly physical impotence had any improvement from these absurd surgical remedies. Thus, until ten years ago, surgery for impotence was a series of fads passed on from one doctor to another without any laboratory investigation or scientific basis. Gullible physicians performed thousands of operations on desperate men who only wanted to be able to have an erection.

The First Successful Operations

The concept of surgically placing a stiff rod of some sort into the penis to create an erection originated in 1936 in Germany. In the initial operations of this type, a section of rib cartilage was placed inside the penis to give it rigidity. The idea behind this first reasonable surgical approach to impotence was that many mammals normally obtain their erection by virtue of a bone in their penis. In the whale this bone is over six feet long and in the walrus it is nearly two feet long. It is much smaller in the bear and the wolf. In most of these mammals the bone is absolutely essential for intercourse to take place. In squirrels it sticks out of the end of the penis and is very sharp. In the otter intercourse is sometimes so violent that the penis fractures and heals many times during the course of an otter's lifetime. Erection in humans and in monkeys is such a remarkably complicated phenomenon that scientists still aren't completely sure exactly how it occurs. A bone acting as an internal splint to guide the penis into the mate's vagina is the usual, simple solution that most animals, aside from humans and monkeys, have found quite acceptable.

The basis of all recent attempts at surgery for impotence has been to find a rod or implant that would create an erection as reliably as in these animals, yet look and feel like a human erection. Unfortunately, the early rib cartilage grafts and plastic rods experimented with until the early 1970s frequently created tissue reaction, became infected, produced pressure defects and discomfort. They rubbed against the tissue compartment in the penis and eventually eroded their way out of it. They were uncomfortable, and usually did not give the same feeling that a normal erection would have.

Then a dramatic improvement came upon the scene in the mid-1970s. A nonreactive, silicone, semirigid rod was developed that gave perfectly normal feeling and performing erections. The most popular implant of this type, called the Small–Carrion prosthesis, was the first that gave "normal" erections to men who were totally impotent and also provided very satisfactory intercourse. The only problem was that the erection was always there, and after the initial excitement over being able to have sex went away, many men asked to have these rods removed because they just didn't like walking around all day long with an erection. To solve this problem, Dr. Roy Finney developed a plastic rod similar to the Small–Carrion except that it had a little hinge on it that allowed the rigid penis to be bent out of the way, making it easier to conceal.

These rods cannot be placed anywhere under the skin of the penis, but must be separately inserted into each of the two cavernous spaces which literally compose the backbone of the penis and which would normally fill with blood during the usual process of erection. These cavernous spaces are enclosed by very strong, dense, ligamentous capsules, which is why they are so impervious to damage despite all sorts of trauma during normal intercourse. If the implants are not positioned within these spaces, the penile skin alone is not able to tolerate the trauma of intercourse, and the rods will eventually erode out. The cavernous spaces extend all the way to the base of the buttocks, just like the foundation of a skyscraper. If the silicone implants did not fill the entire cavernous spaces down to this foundation, the erection would be very unstable and would not support intercourse adequately.

The New Inflatable Erection

The early versions of surgically implanted erection devices had many problems. The greatest difficulty was that they provided the patient with a permanent erection. This could be embarrassing on the beach or at the tennis courts, not to mention at a conservative business meeting. Although we may enjoy intercourse for a brief period during the day or evening, we certainly don't need to have an erection all day long. The new devices have solved this problem in various ways.

Since normal erection in a potent man results from the two cavernous spaces inside the penis literally inflating with blood during sexual arousal, Dr. F. Brantley Scott of Houston in the early

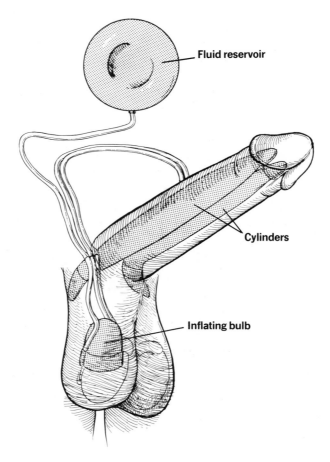

The Inflatable Erection: cylinders inflated to cause erection

1970s decided that the best implant would be inflatable and mimic the natural physiology of erection. With the prosthesis Dr. Scott invented, the patient can produce his own erection at will. He simply activates this device by repeatedly squeezing an inflating bulb in the scrotum which pumps fluid out of a reservoir into two inflatable cylinders, each one implanted in one of the cavernous bodies of the penis. As the prosthesis inflates, so does the penis. After intercourse the patient activates a release valve in the same scrotal pump. This allows fluid to move back out of the penis and

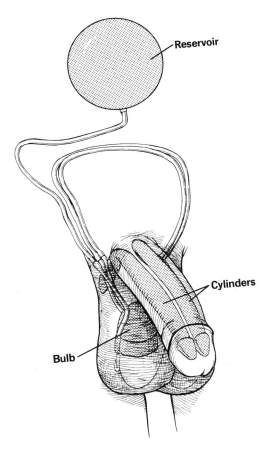

The Inflatable Erection: cylinders deflated during flaccid state

into the reservoir, allowing the penis to once again become limp. This device has been tested in the laboratory and found capable of producing normal erections twice daily for at least twenty years before it is likely to fail. The entire device consists of a reservoir of fluid, a pump to move the fluid, and two inflatable cylinders inserted in the cavernous bodies of the penis, all of these devices connected by tubing and valves. Previous prostheses allowed good sexual intercourse, but left the penis permanently erect. With the inflatable prosthesis, a fairly normal erection is now available to any man with otherwise permanent impotence.

However, the device is not without complications. One patient was so excited that he could have erections that in the first six postoperative weeks he never wanted to deflate it. By keeping his erection permanently inflated, he left the fluid reservoir empty all the time. Scar tissue built up around the reservoir and began to compress it so that finally six weeks later, when he decided he was actually willing to let his erection deflate, he wasn't able to do so. The reservoir was literally encased in contracting scar tissue. Thus, none of the fluid could travel out of the penis.

Although the device is carefully designed not to allow an accidental deflation one can imagine how nerve-racking it would be to suddenly become flaccid in the middle of intercourse because of a fluid leak. Indeed, fluid leaks and kinks in the tubing will occur in about 15 to 20 percent of patients, requiring an additional operation either to correct the kink or to repair the leakage. With the exception of these problems, 95 percent of the patients are very happy with the outcome of this surgery. Thus surgery for impotence finally seems to be emerging from an era of ignorance, superstition, and unscientific methodology. If part of this chapter seems humorous or embarrassing, it is only because we are taking an objective overview of one of the male's most important functions. So much emotion and intensity of feeling are tied up in this simple inflation and deflation of the penis that any rational discussion of it sometimes causes a giggle.

8

Pain in the Testicles

There are very few men who have escaped the absolutely miserable sensation of being hit or kicked in the testicles during some athletic event. It is excruciatingly painful and creates an almost inexpressible sense of horror. Equally horrifying is the experience of a sudden unexplained attack of pain and swelling in the testicles. Sometimes that swelling is a sign of an impending catastrophe which, if not operated on immediately, will result in loss of the testicle. It could also be an infection that doesn't threaten the future existence of the testicle, but that could result in sterility if not treated properly. Making the right diagnosis promptly is critically important. It behooves all men, young or old, to understand enough about their testicles that they can recognize when they are in danger.

Torsion, or Twisted Testicle

The testicle floats freely within a small lubricated space in the scrotum. We can tell how mobile the testicles are just by stepping out of a cold swimming pool and seeing how they are drawn close to the body by the cremasteric muscle. When it is cold outside, this muscle pulls the testicles up to keep them warm. When it is hot outside the muscle relaxes, and the testicles descend and cool off. The reason that the testicles are allowed such mobility is that their temperature must be precisely regulated to be at 94° Fahrenheit. If the testicles are allowed to get too warm, they will not make sperm sufficiently. Thus our fertility is preserved by a complex temperature-regulating mechanism that requires that the testicles be highly mobile.

However, that mobility can occasionally be disastrous. The testicle may actually twist around on the cord from which it hangs. This cord contains the blood vessels that nourish the testicle and the vas deferens, which carries sperm from the testicle into the ejaculate. When the testicle twists on its cord, the blood vessels become kinked. Arterial blood can still get into it because it is driven by very high pressure, but blood that should return from the testicle through the veins cannot get out. Thus, the testicle becomes massively swollen. If the testicle is not untwisted within four to eight hours, it will die a slow and agonizing death. Swelling and pain are excruciating for three to five days, and by that time the testicle can easily become the size of a large grapefruit. Then over the next three months the swelling gradually subsides, the testicle shrinks, and by the end of another three months shrivels to the size of a little pea, a ghost of the testicle that has died.

As frightening as this may sound, the diagnosis of torsion is missed in most cases. People who are unfortunate enough to have their testicles twist usually lose them, and most often don't even know why. Patients with suddenly swollen testicles usually get placed on antibiotics under the mistaken notion that the swelling is caused by an infection. The pain and swelling do eventually subside, and the patient is not aware that his testicle has disappeared until three months later. Yet if a simple ten-minute operation to untwist the testicle had been performed immediately, the testicle could have survived.

I recently received a pitiful letter from a twenty-four-year-old man who said, "At age 15 my right testicle swelled to three times normal size. One year later the left one did the same thing. Both have shrunk to the size of a marble. I have gradually been having fewer erections and less sexual desire. I also feel like my sperm has dried up. Do you know anything about this rare problem of mine?"

Why did lightning strike twice in this man, first on one side and then on the other? If he had only lost one testicle from torsion, he would still be a normal man. Why did it happen a year later to the other side, thus making him a eunuch? The reason is that testicles that undergo torsion have an anatomic structural configuration that makes them easily twistable, and this peculiarity is usually present on both sides. Thus, if the diagnosis of twisted testicle is missed and the patient loses his testicle on one side, he is at a very high risk of someday, without warning, losing the other testicle as well. Unfortunately for the man who wrote this letter, neither his doctors nor his parents realized that he should have had a simple operation to fix the other testicle in place with a few stitches so that it would no longer be susceptible to torsion. Had that simple operation been performed, the second testicle would never have twisted and he would not now be a eunuch.

I recently saw a sophisticated young oil executive whose right testicle had swelled up when he was fourteen years of age. He was told that he had an infection called epididymitis. The testicle shrank into nothing three months later, yet nothing was done to protect the other testicle. Three years later, his remaining (left) testicle swelled up, and again he was told that he had epididymitis. The patient really didn't make much of the fact that his testicles had shriveled up and disappeared, because he just assumed that the "infection" had been cured. Then he began to note hot flashes, flushing, and sweating episodes similar to those experienced by women undergoing menopause. He would have at least one such episode about every hour during the day. Doctors who initially saw him after he lost his second and only testicle noted that the patient still obtained erection and that his sexual interest had not altered since his "epididymitis." He was a senior in high school at that time and indeed might never have found out what was wrong if it weren't for the fact that his mother at that time was going through menopause, and she was a nurse. Of course, his erections gradually became less frequent, and his sexual desire dropped off, so that finally three or four years later, he had to be placed on testosterone injections in order to restore his manhood.

He received these shots once every six weeks, and found he had an active interest in sex for the first ten days afterwards, but this then dropped off fairly sharply. The hot flashes developed about five to six weeks after the shots, just before he was due for his next injection. The hair on his chest and his beard would start to grow during the first two weeks after the injection, and then would slow down and fall out during the subsequent four weeks prior to his next shot. After a full year, his doctor realized that he would need to be on these injections every seven to ten days in order to obtain a stable mood, sexual ability, beard, and masculine hair distribution. I finally saw him thirteen years after he had become a eunuch, at the age of thirty. At that time he still did not fully understand what had actually happened to him. An infection like epididymitis would not have caused him to lose both his testicles. If he had had the simple ten-minute operation to untwist and fix his testicles, he would have been spared the misery of having to go through his whole life with hormone replacements.

I have seen many such uninformed patients who have already lost one testicle from torsion sometime in the past, yet have not had their sole remaining testicle fixed in position to prevent it from twisting also. One patient who had lost his right testicle from torsion was actually told that the swelling and the pain were caused by a kidney stone trying to pass!

Epididymitis

"Epididymitis" simply means that the duct work (called the epididymis) that conveys sperm out of the testicle into the vas deferens is inflamed and swollen. Usually this is caused by bacteria migrating from the urinary tract, backwards, through the vas deferens, down toward the testicle. Epididymitis is extremely common. Almost any man who has ever had prostate troubles has a very good chance of someday getting epididymitis. The bacteria that cause this swelling normally reside in many men, but usually cause no trouble. These bacteria are very difficult for many laboratories to culture and identify. Epididymitis can cause a tremendous amount of swelling in the scrotum that is often very difficult, if not impossible, to distinguish from torsion. Yet epididymitis should never be operated on, and torsion should always be operated on. Epididymitis simply requires large doses of antibiotics and antiinflammatory drugs, but torsion requires an untwisting operation, So if a man's testicle suddenly swells up and begins to hurt, he is in a real dilemma. The doctor must be able to determine promptly whether the swelling is caused by infection or whether the testicle is twisted. A proper decision can mean the difference between remaining a normal man and becoming a eunuch.

There are several clues to whether the diagnosis is epididymitis or torsion, but following them dogmatically can be disastrous. In men under the age of twenty a swollen testicle is most commonly caused by twisting, and over the age of twenty it is most commonly caused by epididymitis. If there is infection in the urine, the testicle swelling is most likely to be epididymitis, and if there is no infection in the urine, it is most likely to be torsion. Unfortunately, these guidelines are so riddled with exceptions that if we relied on them many adults over the age of twenty would lose their testicles and many children under the age of twenty would undergo unnecessary surgery and, more important, perhaps not have prompt antibiotic treatment. If epididymitis is not treated promptly, it can result in scarring of the sperm duct so that even though the patient has not lost his tesicles or his manhood, the sperm cannot get out and he will be infertile.

Luckily there are now two simple methods for making the correct diagnosis in virtually every case. One involves taking a "nuclear scan" of the scrotum, and the other the use of an instrument called the Doppler stethoscope. Both of these simple techniques tell quickly whether blood is flowing in and out of the testicle properly. If it is, then the testicle is not twisted, and the diagnosis is epididymitis.

The nuclear scan involves injecting a tiny, harmless dose of a radioactive substance called technetium into an arm vein and putting a Geiger-counter-type device over the scrotum. If blood flow to the testicle is adequate, the Geiger counter will detect and record it. The Doppler stethoscope involves a special type of ultrasound sonar device similar to what the Navy uses in its submarines to detect underwater structures. This device consists of a little probe that is placed over the scrotum. If the testicle is receiving normal blood flow, a rapid swishing sound can actually be heard on a loudspeaker attached to the stethoscope. This indicates that the testicle is not twisted and, again, that the diagnosis is epididymitis. If no pulsatile swishing sound is heard, it means that the testicle is twisted and needs to be untwisted.

I recently had a call from a pediatrician whose fourteen-year-old boy had suddenly developed severe left-sided scrotal pain and swelling. Because the child was under twenty, it seemed likely that he had torsion, requiring immediate surgery. But rather than jump to that conclusion, we listened first with the Doppler stethoscope and heard normal arterial pulsation. In fact, the pulsations were even louder on the swollen side, indicating inflammation. We then also did the scrotal nuclear scan and found normal radioactive counts in the testicle, indicating good blood flow. The child thus avoided unnecessary surgery and was able to receive prompt antibiotic treatment, which hopefully has prevented the scarring that could have caused him to be sterile as an adult.

But epididymitis more typically occurs in men over twenty. I recently saw a man who had already lost his right testicle at age twelve from torsion. Suddenly at age forty-nine his left testicle swelled up to four times its normal size, and he had difficulty urinating. Because of previous torsion on the right side, we might have been very suspicious that his only remaining testicle might now be twisting thirty-seven years later. In fact, his urinalysis showed infection, the Doppler stethoscope demonstrated normal arterial pulsations, and the scrotal nuclear scan showed good blood flow. We therefore didn't have to operate, but rather placed him promptly on antibiotics. The man had a typical history of prostate infection over the previous ten years, and it was predictable that he had a very good chance of one day thus clobbering his epididymis.

Hydrocoele

There is one common sort of scrotal swelling that should not be as worrisome as epididymitis or torsion. The lubricated space in which the testicle floats freely is called the hydrocoele sac. When a testicle twists due to torsion, it is doing so within this lubricated sac. This sac is a vestige of the internal abdominal lining that pouches through the abdomen when someone has a hernia. All men have hydrocoele sacs. But what doctors think of as a "hydrocoele" requiring treatment is when this lubricated space becomes overfilled with lubricating fluid. When this happens, the scrotum looks swollen and some men with this condition think they've got big testicles. They worry that tumor, infection, or all sorts of terrible things may be happening to their testicle. But it is not their testicle that is bigger. It is simply this fluid-filled space that their testicle resides in that is bigger.

When children have a hydrocoele, it is virtually always associated with a hernia. In such cases, the internal abdominal lining never quite closed off at the groin area when the testicle originally came down from the abdomen during the child's embryonic growth in his mother's womb. Thus abdominal fluid is continually leaking through this channel into the scrotum. However, when a middle-aged or older man has a hydrocoele, it is rarely part of a hernia, but simply represents an unexplained accumulation of too much lubricating fluid in this enlarging sac. The condition is harmless, but can be aggravating and irritating. Most people request surgery to correct it. In a child the surgery must involve an incision in the groin rather than the scrotum in order to close off the hernia. In an adult it simply involves a scrotal incision and opening the sac so that the lubricating fluid can no longer get trapped.

Mumps

It might seem that if bacteria can leak down through the sperm ducts, causing epididymitis and a swollen scrotum, it should be able to continue traveling into the testicle. In fact, bacteria usually stop at the epididymitis and do not usually infect the testicle. The reason is that there are valves between the epididymis and the testicle that allow sperm to flow forward out of the testicle but do not allow bacteria to flow backward into the testicle. Thus a man can have the most terrible infection in the scrotum, causing an enormous amount of swelling of the epididymis, but no testicular damage.

On the other hand, there are some infections that do get into the testicle. The most common is mumps. The mumps virus does not flow backward from the urine through the sperm duct into the epididymis, but is disseminated throughout the bloodstream, and for some reason, in postpubertal males only, it frequently lodges in the testicle. The testicle becomes terribly swollen and painful, and there is nothing that the doctors can do for it. There is a 50 percent chance that the testicle's sperm-producing ability will be destroyed when a man gets the mumps. For some unknown reason, the mumps virus will not attack the testicles of children, but only adults or postpubertal teenagers. Thus it is better to have already had mumps, or vaccination for mumps, during the prepubertal years. Fortunately, mumps usually attacks only one side, but when it attacks both sides, you are very likely to become sterile as a result.

Psychological Pain in the Testicles

Sometimes pain in the testicles can result from psychological causes. In such cases, the origin of the pain cannot be determined, though the patient's misery is real.

I recently received a letter from a man who said he had had a problem with his right testicle for the past two years. "I have had constant pain and I can only get through a day's work by taking pain relievers. I have been going to doctors ever since the problem started. I have seen some of the best urologists . . . I have had nerve blocks done also but only received minor relief for a few hours." The patient had absolutely nothing detectably wrong with his testicle. Yet he was convinced that there was something wrong, and such a patient will often go through one operation after another, dividing nerves, blocking nerves, and even removing part of the epididymis, but always to no avail, except perhaps to make the pain worse.

Sometimes testicular pain is truly in the testicle, and not in the head, but it can be very difficult to distinguish. The only clue to the psychological nature of this pain is that it frequently wanders all over the genitalia, even into the abdomen, and sometimes down into the rectum, with no regard for the normal nerve pathways and anatomical configuration. A typical example is a patient recently referred to me from a leading medical institution in the East after he had seen many urologists. His problem began after a vasectomy. He wrote to me, "Pain and sexual dysfunction have persisted to this day. Treatment has consisted of antibiotics, anti-inflammatory drugs and nerve blocks. Darvon is needed even now to get out of bed. Sexual problems exist, and touching the scrotum especially on the left side elicits pain. Ejaculation is painful and premature, followed by severe aching in the lower abdomen, scrotum, and prostate areas. Each night erections have been experienced while in a deep sleep which refuse to subside unless I get out of bed and stand up." (These erections during sleep we know are normal.) His pain migrated around without any regard to known anatomy. He could not deal with his sterility, and was only expressing his fear and frustration. Doctors can be so confused by these bizarre pains in the genitals that they are often tempted to prescribe one drug after another, or even try surgery, just to get the patient off their back.

Whenever men are plagued by weird fantasies about their genitalia, their explanations tend to be long and laborious. In fact, that is the doctor's immediate clue that their problem is mental rather than physical. At the end of a detailed five-page letter, one man concluded, "My sexual life is impaired, my meditative life is threatened and I feel hindered from trying to heal myself. If you could help to bring my right testicle back to a state of health you would change my life completely. The urologist said that the spermatic cord is not broken but something is wrong during orgasm. It is as if electrical currents were broken or passages of the back of the testicle blocked. The right testicle seems to work slower, to recover vigor slower after intercourse than the left, and to produce less of the fluids and whatever other fluids that might circulate into the body."

It is this kind of detailed explanation and rationalization that represents the all too excessive introspection that men may have about their genitals. A man can't function well if he is thinking that much about it. It creates imaginary pain that sometimes seems intensely real, and prevents joyful, thoughtless, blissful sexual activity.

9

The Prostate Gland

Why Does the Prostate Cause So Much Trouble?

One male organ which eventually goes wrong in all men is the prostate gland. The prostate gland is located just below the bladder and sits around the outlet of the bladder like a doughnut, and we begin our urination through the doughnut hole. The purpose of the prostate gland is to produce the fluid called semen that transports sperm out into the ejaculate. The prostate gland is tiny in prepubertal boys, but at the time of puberty grows to about the size of a nickel in diameter. As men get older, particularly over the age of forty, the prostate begins to grow again inexorably, so that it can sometimes be quite large by the time they are in their sixties or seventies (possibly even as large as a grapefruit). This gradual enlargement of the prostate with aging seems to result from a slow change in the hormonal environment produced by the testicles. Castrated men never get this enlargement of the prostate. It depends upon the hormones produced by the testicle. This inevitable enlargement of the prostate with age is called benign prostatic hypertrophy. It is not cancer.

As the prostate enlarges, the hole in its center becomes

smaller. The enlarging bulk of the prostate gland spreads inward as well as outward, and tightens around the urethra, thereby slowing or cutting off the flow of urine. Thus, as men get older and the prostate gets larger, the passageway through which the urine is pushed out of the bladder gets smaller and smaller, and the bladder has to work harder and harder. The bladder muscles thicken and bundle up into contracted, spastic fibers, much like the muscles of a weight lifter, in order to build up the power necessary to force the urine out of this shrinking hole.

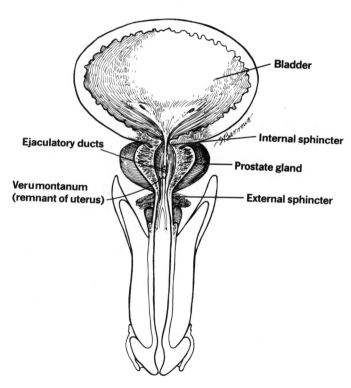

The Prostate Gland

The first sign of the prostate's enlargement is when a man has to urinate more often than usual. He is more likely to notice this problem during the night, when he may have to start getting up from sleep once or twice to urinate. Eventually this may progress to the point where he is getting up three or four times a night. He won't usually make that much urine, but he still has an intense need to urinate. Despite this urgency, he may not be *able* to urinate immediately. This is called hesitancy. After waiting in line in a public bathroom at the movie house or the football game, instead of emptying his bladder immediately, he may notice that he has to stand there embarrassingly, agonizingly, as long as twenty to thirty seconds before he finally gets his stream started. Then after he's finished urinating he may find that some of the urine continues to dribble, often wetting the pants. He may notice that the force of his stream steadily gets weaker as he gets older. All men remember how easy it would be in their early years to write their name in the snow while urinating. But very few men over the age of forty can boast of that skill. Eventually if a man is very unlucky he may one day find that he cannot urinate at all, and have to be rushed to the hospital to have a catheter put in to drain his bladder.

There are three basic problems of the prostate gland. One is this benign prostatic hypertrophy, which occurs in all men as they get older, but seems worse for some than others. Another is prostatitis, a very common infection of the prostate gland that occurs in a large number of men between the ages of twenty-five and fifty. Finally, there is cancer of the prostate, the second most common cancer among men in the United States. Cancer of the prostate also seems to be an inevitable result of aging. Eighty percent of men at the age of eighty have cancer in their prostate gland, as do 15 percent of men over the age of fifty. But the vast majority of these cancers are biologically nonaggressive, asymptomatic, not even detectable clinically, and will never harm the patient. In fact, despite the fact that 80 percent of men over the age of eighty have cancer of the prostate, not very many of them die of that disease. Most of these men die of heart disease before this extremely slow-growing and biologically nonaggressive cancer becomes lethal. Yet when it is aggressive, it is a deadly, tragic condition.

Prostatitis

Prostatitis is perhaps the most common condition seen by urologists. Patients with prostatitis are typically too young to have undergone the hypertrophy, or growth, of the prostate gland that occurs in men over the age of forty. Prostatitis is an inflammation, probably an infection, that does not seem to be venereal in origin. It is amazing that this common problem still defies any good explanation as to what causes it. The debates in medical circles about this condition are legion. In perhaps 5 percent of the cases bacteria can be cultured from either the urine or from prostatic fluid obtained by massage, but in the vast majority of cases no clearly identifiable bacteria can be cultured. The evidence that some kind of bacteria is responsible for prostatitis is circumstantial, yet compelling, based upon the fact that despite the absence of any proof of a bacterial cause, most people with prostatitis get better with long-term tetracycline antibiotic treatment.

It seems certain that whatever it is that causes prostatitis is not transferred venereally. In fact, infrequent sexual activity seems more likely to cause prostatitis than frequent or varied sexual activity. For some reason the typical patient with prostatitis is someone who has irregular sexual activity rather than a regular two to three times a week program. It used to be called the "sailor's disease." After being out to sea for six months, when they came into port some sailors would have sex three or four times a day for several days, and then go back out to sea for another six months. For some reason or other, sporadic bursts of sexual activity in between long episodes of abstinence are most likely to lead to severe and acute attacks of prostatitis. Many doctors tell their patients who are having sex infrequently to simply have more sex in an effort to stave off the prostatitis. But it isn't how much sex a man has or how little he has, but merely the regularity of intervals of sex.

An acute attack of prostatitis is a frightfully uncomfortable condition. Besides having to urinate frequently, ejaculation is extremely painful, as is urination. It doesn't just burn at the tip (as in urethritis), but deep at the base of the penis. There is a swollen feeling around the base of the penis that is hard to describe because there is no visible swelling. It is deep within. Frequently there are fever, chills, and systemic signs of infection. The doctor may see a very small number of red blood cells in the urine, but rarely does the urinalysis show anything else.

In the more chronic types of prostatitis, the patient may not have this sudden, severe pain and difficulty urinating, but rather he may simply notice that he has to go to the bathroom more frequently, probably several times during the night, that his stream is weaker, and that it takes somewhat longer to get it started.

Perhaps these attacks of nonspecific prostatitis are caused by an accumulation of the secretions of the prostate gland that aren't being released by a regular interval of ejaculation. But regardless of the interpretation of what causes this extraordinarily common and yet mysterious disease, high doses of long-term tetracycline seem to control most of the cases. There may be frequent recurrences, and some of the symptoms may persist, but basically most patients are relieved of most of their symptoms with this particular antibiotic. It is rare that any kind of surgery would ever be recommended for this condition.

Benign Prostatic Hypertrophy

Growth of the prostate is an inevitable consequence of aging, and no man can escape it. It is usually a benign condition, and there is no cause for a man to worry that he is suffering from malignancy. The frequent, tiny focuses of cancer of the prostate do not account for this remarkable enlargement. Antibiotics will not cure the symptoms of an enlarging prostate. Only surgery to remove it will rid one of the symptoms. But such surgery is usually not recommended until one is somewhat older, because most people can live with the symptoms for some time. When the symptoms really become aggravating and threaten the ability to urinate, then a procedure called transurethral prostatectomy (TUR) is usually recommended sometime in the patient's sixties or seventies.

In the past this operation was frequently done through a large abdominal incision and sometimes under a general anesthetic. The mortality rate was extremely high. In fact, forty years ago the mortality rate from this procedure was so high that prostatism was considered very very deadly. Subject a seventy-year-old man with other health problems to a large abdominal incision, in which there is a lot of bleeding, and it is understandable that the operation could be dangerous. But with modern techniques a little telescope is placed up through the penis and the prostate is literally scraped out in a methodical fashion without any incision being made. This way there is very little pain, very little splinting of the muscles of breathing because of this pain, and the whole procedure can be done under a spinal anesthetic with little trauma to the patient, who is often too old to tolerate a gigantic surgical undertaking. Thus, what used to be a dreaded and a painful surgical condition that was put off as long as possible is now relatively painless, with hospitalization for no more than several days.

But even this more modern operation, the TUR, must be performed carefully, and only by a surgeon very experienced in it because it is not just a matter of scraping out tissue. The prostate can bleed tremendously, and it is easy for the surgeon to lose sight of landmarks through the telescope if he is not experienced. He could even inadvertently damage the sphincter that controls urination, and there can be nothing more miserable for a man than dripping urine all the time because his sphincter has been damaged by an inaccurately performed prostatectomy.

A normal consequence of the operation is that afterward

there is no longer any fluid coming out in the ejaculate. Patients who have undergone this surgery say that their sensation of orgasm and ejaculation is just as pleasurable, but the sperm simply go backward into the bladder rather than forward out the penis. This operation does not remove *all* of the prostate gland. It is the inner core of the prostate that is removed, leaving the outer shell undisturbed. In fact, the outer shell represents the true prostate that has been there all along. Once the inner pulp has been removed, urination is dramatically easier and once again a man can write his name in the snow as he could when he was a little boy.

Cancer of the Prostate

Cancer of the prostate is an incredibly common disease. If men live long enough, they will nearly all get it. But before worrying about this inevitable cancer that attacks the genitals, the male should remember that, as we said earlier, in the vast majority of cases these cancers are not biologically active, produce no symptoms, are extremely tiny in comparison with the rest of the gland, and do not grow or cause death.

At least 10 percent of men undergoing TUR or prostatectomy for benign prostatic hypertrophy have a little focus of cancer. Autopsy specimens of the prostate gland in men who died of other causes show cancer in as many as 10 percent of men between the ages of fifty and fifty-nine, 30 percent of men between ages sixty and sixty-nine, and over 80 percent of men beyond the age of eighty. So it is clear that most of these clinically undetectable cancers of the prostate never progress into significant disease.

Yet 17,000 men die of cancer of the prostate every year in the United States, and it is a leading cause of cancer deaths among American men. These 17,000 deaths are a small number when compared to the literally millions of men who are walking around with clinically undetectable prostate cancer. Still it is obvious that some of these cancers can start growing and can kill.

The problem is how to detect which cancers of the prostate need treatment and which can be left alone. If doctors simply wait until the cancer becomes clinically detectable without screening tests, the majority of patients will be beyond cure by the time the cancer is discovered. In fact, 50 percent of prostatic cancers that become clinically detectable have already spread to all regions of the body. Furthermore, close to 40 percent of tumors have spread beyond the confines of the prostate. Thus only a small fraction of prostate cancers that become clinically detectable other than through a massive screening program have a very good chance of cure. Although doctors certainly do not want to go on a witch hunt for cancer of the prostate, which they know is eventually going to be found in millions upon millions of American men and do no harm, nonetheless they are in a quandary. If they sit back and wait for these tumors to appear, by the time they do most of them will have already gotten beyond the stage where cure is possible. The symptoms of urinary distress are caused almost always by benign prostatic enlargement or prostatitis, but the early cancer of the prostate, which is potentially curable, has no symptoms. The most common and best method of diagnosing cancer of the prostate is for the urologist to do a rectal exam.

One general rule that doctors have found useful is that prostate cancer is most likely to grow and spread beyond the prostate (i.e., behave like cancer) if there are several focuses diffusely located throughout the prostate gland, or if the one focus is large enough to represent a palpable lump. So when such a cancer is discovered incidentally at the time of a TUR or a routine rectal examination, the doctors are aggressive in treating it. But in the vast majority of cases a single focus of prostate cancer requires no treatment.

When a cancer is detected that does require treatment (and has a chance for surgical cure), the type of prostatectomy performed is not the common operation used for men with benign prostatic hypertrophy. In cancer cases the entire prostate gland is removed, not just the inner pulp and core. This results in a discontinuity between the bladder and the urinary tube, the urethra. So the surgeon then sews the bladder back to the urinary tube. The prostate is now entirely out of the picture. This radical removal of the prostate for cancer creates impotence in every case, and has about a 10 to 20 percent chance of leaving the patient with uncontrollable urinary leakage. So radical surgery for prostate cancer is not to be undertaken lightly. Remember that surgery for benign prostatic enlargement, which only removes the inner core, should *not* cause impotence or urinary leakage.

Before a prostate cancer is removed in this fashion, most surgeons perform staging operations to find out whether the cancer has already spread to lymph nodes outside of the prostate. They would not want to subject their patients to total, radical prostatectomy if the tumor has already escaped into nearby areas. Thus very often the pelvic lymph nodes are first removed through an operation in the lower abdomen to determine whether there is any chance for cure of the prostate cancer. Whether or not lymph nodes are involved, radiation is sometimes used either as a replacement for surgery or in addition to surgery to enhance its effectiveness.

What about the man whose prostate cancer has spread throughout the body? This constitutes at least 50 percent of patients who turn up with clinically detectable prostate cancer. Has he no hope for cure? Thanks to an absolutely miraculous discovery in 1941 by Dr. Charles Huggins, a urologist who received the Nobel Prize in medicine for this work, we know that 80 percent of these prostate cancers, no matter how widespread, are dependent on the male hormone testosterone for their continued growth. The minute the body stops making testosterone, tumors that are on the verge of killing the patient disappear almost magically and quite instantaneously. Patients who appeared to be on their deathbed, in miserable pain, and nearly comatose, will after castration improve overnight, wake up the next day bright and cheerful, and go home within the week. The most remarkable sensation in my whole life was as a third-year medical student on the urology service when I saw a man in the final throes of stage D prostate cancer brought to the VA

Hospital. He appeared almost dead. The urologist performed a simple castration procedure, and literally overnight the patient revived, and one week later he was walking around the ward joking with everybody and anxious to go home.

Castration is a dramatic way to cure these patients, but another way to achieve the same effect is to give them the female hormone, estrogen. This female hormone depresses their pituitary gland's ability to make the hormone that stimulates testosterone production by the testicle. So the administration of estrogen is a pharmacological way of performing castration.

It is fortunate that so many of these advanced prostate cancers are dependent on testosterone for their very survival, and that as soon as the supply of this hormone is stopped, the cancer cells shrink and die. However, in most cases, several years later (usually from five to ten years later), small subpopulations of cancer cells that were not dependent on testosterone slowly begin to multiply in the sites where previous tumors had disappeared. So most patients who have had a remission after castration or estrogen can expect their tumor sooner or later to recur, if they live long enough. But in the meantime they've had many extra years of life because of this remarkable discovery for which the Nobel Prize was justly awarded many years ago.

PART THREE
The Little Boy's Problems

10
Circumcision

Is It a Good Idea?

The first worry a man will ever have about his genitals occurs immediately after birth, when he undergoes circumcision, and he has no part in the decision. For forty thousand years circumcision has been performed by various primitive societies and cultures around the world. Is it a good idea?

All societies, whether primitive or sophisticated, develop a set of rituals that are practiced at the occurrence of certain critical transitions in the life of an individual. When I worked in Australia I spent some time in the center of that vast country and became friendly with several aborigines. These people had a forty-thousand-year-old culture that seemed to work quite well, even though some of their practices are unfathomable to contemporary societies. As I hiked through the desert country with one aboriginal fellow I came to know well, I was fascinated by his quick intelligence and his uncanny ability to find water, food, and literally anything one needed for living in that arid desert that seemed to me so inhospitable. Yet he could not rationally explain to me why it was beneficial to him to have one of his upper front teeth missing—the tooth having been banged out during a ceremony of manhood—or what possible genital advantage his subincision (a modified aboriginal version of circumcision) could have conferred. Yet he wore these features with great pride and a feeling that to have all his teeth and an unmarked penis would be unthinkable.

Circumcision has been ritualistically practiced by an enormously wide variety of primitive as well as advanced peoples throughout the history of the world, in Asia, Africa, North America and South America, Europe, Australia, and Polynesia. The Phoenicians, the Arabs, and perhaps even the Jews originally derived this practice from the ancient Egyptians. It occurs among various tribes of Africa, the Australian aborigines, the Malays of Borneo, the North American and South American Indians, the ancient Aztecs, the Mayas, the Caribs, the Fijians, and the Samoans. However, with the exception of Jews and a small number of tribes of Africa, circumcision was always used as a manhood or pubertal rite, often as an immediate prerequisite to mating and marriage.

It was only the Jews, a few Arabic groups, and a few other scattered tribes that practiced circumcision on the newborn male infant. Since cancer of the penis later in adult life is prevented only by circumcision in infancy, and not by circumcision at any other time, such as puberty, these groups may have had some very special insight. In fact, the multiple origins of circumcision in primitive societies all over the world, societies that could not have possibly had any contact with each other, force us to conclude that despite the primitive and barbaric nature of this ritual there were some obvious health benefits.

Some of the very ancient matriarchal religions that were the immediate precursors of the more paternalistic monotheism of the Jews were based upon worship of mother goddess figures. These religions sometimes required the sacrificial offering of extirpated male genitals to the goddess. In that respect, circumcision may have represented simply a token genital mutilation that satisfied the goddess, but didn't result in the extinction of the tribe as castration would have accomplished.

Jews traditionally view this procedure religiously and perform it as part of a divine contract between God and Abraham. By making this sacrifice to God, the covenant between the children of Israel and the Lord was sealed. The Jewish scholar Maimonides believed that circumcision also had a civilizing effect upon the penis, counteracting excessive lust. The Arabs had begun the practice of circumcision long before the birth of Mohammed, and the Moslem religion in fact does not require circumcision. It is nowhere mentioned in the Koran. Nonetheless, circumcision is traditionally practiced throughout Islam. For Moslems it basically has hygienic and purification connotations and was not originally religious. To Jews it was originally religious, but now has hygienic and purification connotations as well.

There are a number of reasons why circumcision is beneficial and why it ought best be performed in infancy. First, as was said earlier, it prevents cancer of the penis in later life. In a recent study at the University of Puerto Rico, of 500 patients with cancer of the penis, 408 were uncircumcised. The remaining 92 patients had been circumcised, but all of them *after* the newborn period, and two-thirds in adulthood. Cancer of the penis generally occurs when there has been carelessness in taking care of one's foreskin, but a man can be just about as unclean as he likes if he has been circumcised.

Cancer of the penis is a very rare disease and represents only 0.4 percent of all cancer in men in the United States. Yet the various other lesions that frequently occur on the penis that may look similar to cancer are very common. Cancer of the penis is so devastating and terrifying, even for those who survive, and the lesions that look like cancer are so common, that eliminating the risk of cancer of the penis is a benefit not to be taken lightly.

A second benefit of circumcision is that the wives of circumcised men are less commonly afflicted with cancer of the cervix (the opening to the woman's womb). There is controversy currently among doctors on whether it is circumcision that protects against cancer of the cervix, or whether it is some other aspect of hygiene in circumcised men that is responsible. Regardless of the reason, these women are much less likely to suffer the most frequent cancer of the female organs.

The most common benefit of circumcision is that it prevents accumulation of oils and secretions (called smegma) under the foreskin, which lead to infection, swelling, and sometimes contraction of the foreskin so the tip of the penis is trapped inside. Of course, at birth the foreskin normally does not retract. In a normal newborn baby boy the naïve mother might be horrified to find that the foreskin so covers the tip of her boy's penis that there is no way she can pull it back to see if it is normal. Thus many mothers, and even some doctors, will say that the child has a phimosis, an obstructed foreskin, *requiring* circumcision. The mother then figures that it may be very important to have this foreskin removed because her child has a problem with it. Nothing could be further from the truth. Gradually with growth, and eventually adulthood, the foreskin in almost all young boys begins to retract normally as long as it is kept clean. But if the child is not kept clean and if as he grows up he tends not to bathe enough, secretions can become entrapped and cause the foreskin to scar so that he indeed does have a problem. But if he was circumcised in infancy, he will never have to worry about any of this.

Despite its benefits, however, circumcision can cause problems. The primary function of the foreskin in childhood is to protect the tip of the penis, called the glans. Particularly in the young child, when the penis may be in contact with a urine-soaked diaper, smelling of ammonia, the foreskin protects the little opening of the penis, or meatus, from scarring and obstructing proper urination. In fact, one of the most common problems of the penis that urologists see in their pediatric practice is called meatal stenosis. This is when there is a pinpointlike opening instead of the normal slit at the end of the penis, which restricts the flow of urine. This meatal stenosis would rarely be seen in an uncircumcised child, but in a circumcised one it is common, and the reason is that he did not have the protective benefit of a foreskin. Treatment of this pinholelike meatal stenosis is to enlarge the opening surgically (by an operation called meatotomy), but sometimes the opening just scars right down again, and the child may even develop a forked stream, which means that half of the urine goes into the toilet, and half goes onto his shoes.

Circumcision is basically a very safe procedure, but it is not without occasional disaster. When I was a first-year resident in urology I received a call from a rather nervous nurse in the neonatal nursery unit. There had been five children born several days earlier that she wanted me to take a look at, but she would not explain the problem over the phone. When I got to the nursery she explained to me that a new pediatric resident had just rotated onto their service and the day before had performed the usual circumcisions on newborn babies. He had mentioned nothing to anybody on the staff to indicate that any problems had occurred or that he was aware of any problems, but the nurse noted that morning that none of those five children had very much penis left.

Unfortunately, this is a procedure considered to be so simple and relatively unimportant in the medical world that frequently the least experienced doctors are sent in to do it. Furthermore, if they appear shy or hesitant to perform such an operation without any prior training, they may suffer some ridicule for asking help. That is what happened in this case. I must add that the particular doctor involved was a nice fellow who simply didn't realize the gravity of what he had done. Luckily, with plastic surgery, the penises of all of these children eventually healed without any deformities sufficiently severe to mar their later life. Such accidents are rare, fortunately, but those few that do occur indicate the importance of treating this seemingly harmless ritual of male infancy with some respect. The procedure is considered so much a part of our folk ritual and so simple an event that the definitive, three-volume textbook of urology, in which every aspect of complicated penile reconstructive surgery is discussed, makes no mention of the circumcision procedure at all.

How the Circumcision Is Done

For the newborn infant the operation is really fairly simple. Although it must be very painful, the child is traditionally not given an anesthetic because the risk of doing so would be too great. Furthermore, most medical authorities feel that the brief pain caused by the operation has no harmful effect on the child. He can be completely immobilized on a special little circumcision table and not move around. All the doctor really is concerned about is that the child not wiggle and thereby make his job more dangerous. One of the advantages of performing circumcision in infants rather than in older children is that an anesthetic, with all its risks, is not necessary to keep him still during the procedure.

The foreskin is essentially just an extension of the outer penile skin that is redundant and extends well beyond the actual tip of the penis. It is this extra skin that is removed during a circumcision. For the newborn infant a device such as a clamp or a plastic bell is inserted inside the foreskin and around the tip. The foreskin is then cut circumferentially around the clamp. The clamp or the bell is kept in place for a minute or so afterward, crushing all of the tissue along the cut edge that might otherwise bleed. Thus the usual surgical technique of stopping individual bleeders is not necessary. This simple clamp arrangement would not work in older children, which is another reason for performing circumcision within the first week of life.

There is one clamp technique for circumcision, called the guillotine approach, which can appear very frightening. In this procedure the foreskin is pulled and stretched far beyond the tip of the penis and then clamped in guillotine fashion and literally chopped off. To the watching parents it would appear that the tip of the child's penis is being cut off, but of course that isn't what is happening. After the procedure is completed, the foreskin is retracted and the frightened parents can see that the child's penis has been unharmed.

After the circumcision there is always a raw area between

the glans (i.e., the tip) and the skin of the shaft of the penis. This can look rather frightening and give the parents the impression that something terrible has happened to their little boy's penis. Sometimes this raw area bleeds, frightening them even more. Neither the raw area nor the bleeding need really alarm them, because after a week the raw tissue will gradually be covered with skin that migrates from the cut edges, and the area will heal uneventfully.

The operation is much more involved and painful for an adult than for a newborn boy. So if a male is going to be circumcised, he would be wise to have it done before he leaves the hospital nursery. It is intriguing that very few urologists have any experience doing infant circumcisions. Circumcision is probably the most common operation performed in the United States, yet it is performed only by pediatricians and obstetricians. The urologist, the so-called expert on the male organs, would only do a circumcision when an older child or an adult is involved.

11
Hidden Testicles

Most men have two normal testicles in their scrotum. But oddly enough, during most of the fetus's development inside the mother's womb, its testicles are not located anywhere near the scrotum, but rather are high in the abdomen just underneath the kidneys. About one month prior to birth, the testicles begin to journey downward to the scrotum. If the testicles don't make that journey to the scrotum in the last month of the mother's pregnancy, serious problems result. Over 3 percent of newborn boys have just such an empty scrotum. Every year that the testicles are allowed to stay "hidden" in the warmer environment of the abdomen, they deteriorate more and more. In adulthood they will make no sperm, and will eventually even stop making hormone.

Within the first six weeks after conception, while the fetus is still a minute embryo within the womb, the testicle begins as a tiny thickening. It is located in the abdomen exactly where the ovary is located in a female embryo, directly underneath the kidney. The blood vessels that supply the testicle with nourishment therefore come from the kidney region. Then around the final month before birth, the testicle begins its descent into the scrotum. In children that are born prematurely there is a very high incidence of undescended testicle, simply because the child has come out of the womb before the testicle has had a chance to complete its descent into the scrotum.

As the testicle pushes its way out of the abdomen into the scrotum, it passes through what is called the groin region. This is the area where hernias are commonly found in men. A hernia simply means that there is literally a hole in the envelope of the abdomen which contains all the abdominal structures. Sections of bowel can protrude through this hole and come down through the groin into the scrotum. This is what is called a hernia. The reason men can get hernias so easily is that there is always a potential area of weakness at this spot in the lower abdomen where the testicle originally passed into the scrotum. That is why an operation to repair the hernia can sometimes damage the sperm duct or the testicle.

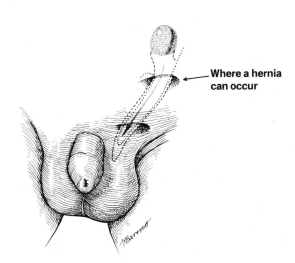

Descent of Testicles from Abdomen into Scrotum

During the testicle's journey through the lower abdominal wall into the scrotum, it naturally encounters the muscular envelope that surrounds the abdomen and pushes a segment of that abdominal muscle in front of it. This scrotal muscle, which is merely a continuation and an out-pouching of the abdominal wall, is called the cremaster muscle. This is the muscle that pulls the testicles close to the body when it is cold outside, and relaxes to allow them to hang low when it is warm out.

This cremaster muscle sometimes may contract so powerfully that it pulls the testicle right back into the abdomen. This so-called "retractile" testicle will descend again when the man relaxes, or when it warms up outside. But it can be very worrisome and very confusing to mothers and children alike when they look for testicles and can't find them. Approximately 6 percent of little boys at one time or other are thought to have undescended testicles, but in the vast majority these are just retractile testes that happen to be hidden in the abdomen because of a very hyperactive cremaster muscle. These retractile testes are completely normal and require no surgery, even though they may spend a good deal of time in the abdomen. They come down enough of the time that their development is normal and surgery is certainly not warranted.

If when the baby is first born the testis is not located in the scrotum, it may very well come down into the scrotum during the next three weeks, just as it would if the baby were still spending that time in the womb. Premature babies frequently have undescended testicles that eventually descend into the scrotum without requiring surgery. However, by the time the infant is three to four months of age, if the testicle has not come into the scrotum yet, it will probably never do so without surgery. About 3 percent of baby boys have no testicles in their scrotum at the time of birth. Yet by three or four months of age, only 0.7 percent still fail to have their testicles normally in place.

In 3 to 5 percent of so-called true undescended testicles there is no testicle at all. If this problem is only present on one side, the child will still grow up to be a normal man. But if he has no testicle on either side, then he will need hormone replacements or a testicle transplant at some time in the future. But luckily 95 percent of boys who have an empty scrotum really do have normal testicles located somewhere in the abdomen, and these can be surgically brought down into the scrotum where they belong.

Why do the testicles have to be in the scrotum? Why can't they remain safely tucked away in the abdomen as the ovaries do in women? The ovaries do not have to be cool in order to function properly, but the testicles do. The testicles simply cannot function properly unless they are four degrees lower in temperature than the rest of the body (i.e., about 94 degrees Fahrenheit). In fact, there is a very intricate cooling mechanism that maintains the testicles' temperature at precisely the required level. The artery that conveys blood and nourishment to the testicle (called the spermatic artery) runs all the way down from the abdomen through the groin and into the testicle. Coiled around this artery is the spermatic vein which returns blood to the abdomen from the testicle. It is coiled around the artery just like a radiator coil in any conventional heating or cooling system. Thus the blood that returns from the scrotum (and which therefore is much cooler than the blood coming to the testicle from the abdomen) is continually circulating around the incoming spermatic artery. That is, the chilly blood leaving the scrotum cools the warm blood entering the scrotum, thereby maintaining the required testicular temperature. This can only work if the testicle is located outside of the body in a separately cooled scrotal sac.

When the testicle is located in the abdomen, it cannot make sperm at all, and even the production of male hormone (which is much more resilient) eventually slows down earlier in life than it should. Thus any man whose testicles remain in the abdomen is surely sterile, and though he may have normal male characteristics and normal male sex drive in his youth, they tend to deteriorate as he reaches his late thirties or forties.

I had a twenty-one-year-old patient several years ago who had just gotten married, and decided with his wife that it might be patriotic for the two of them to enlist simultaneously in the military to pursue a career together. He was a normal fellow with a good sex life and normal aspirations for a family. His wife was immediately accepted for military service, but he was rejected because the examining officer discovered that there were no testicles in his scrotum. This came as a bit of a shock because he had had regular pediatric examinations as a child, and thought of himself as being a perfectly normal man with a normal penis and a normal sex life.

His testicles could not produce sperm anymore because of this long-neglected problem, but they were obviously still making male hormone. Thus he had gone through the normal pubertal changes of manhood. But if his testicles remained in the abdomen, they would eventually be totally destroyed. He would then undergo a premature drop in hormone production as he got older, and literally become a castrate.

It is ironic that he was not accepted for military duty because he had no testicles, but his wife was accepted for military duty even though she had no testicles either. It seemed a bit unfair.

Another final caution to men who may notice that there are no testicles in their scrotum is that these abdominal testicles are much more prone to developing cancer than are normal ones. In fact, cancer of the testicle is forty to fifty times more frequent in men whose testicles have not descended. Surgery to bring the testicles into the scrotum may improve sperm production and protect the testicles from premature hormonal decline, but it will not protect them from the increased risk of developing cancer. Testicle cancer normally occurs in about two out of every hundred thousand men, but in men with undescended testicles the risk of cancer is one in a thousand. So the risk is still low, even though it is fifty times normal. If the testicles are surgically brought into the scrotum, at least they can be examined frequently, so that if a tumor should develop, it can be detected early enough for a high probability of cure. For this reason as well, it is important not to let testicles remain hidden.

In the majority of cases surgery to bring the testicle into the scrotum is relatively simple. When the testicle is located low in the abdomen, it is a simple matter of freeing it from surrounding tissue and transferring it into the scrotum. However, in some cases the testicle is so high in the abdomen that the surgery is incredibly delicate and fraught with a great risk of losing the testicle completely. In such cases, the testicle cannot be brought into the scrotum with ordinary surgical techniques. Instead, the blood vessels that are nourishing it have to be completely detached and then reconnected to blood vessels closer to the scrotum. This is the so-called testicle autotransplant. Because the testicular blood vessels are so very tiny, the reconnection has to be performed under a microscope with stitches that are essentially invisible to the naked eye. This sort of testicle microvascular autotransplant has to be performed on about 5 percent of boys who have undescended testicles. In most such cases, the surgeon is not equipped to perform this kind of operation, and the testicles may be easily damaged or lost completely.

It is very easy for a physician to casually suggest that such high testicles be removed rather than perform the difficult surgery of autotransplanting them into the scrotum. But it is the patient who has to live with the irregular hormone levels and painful injections associated with lifelong testosterone replacement. Such a decision is too important to be left in the physician's hands. The patient and his parents must simply know the alternatives and the risks and be allowed to make the decision for themselves. In almost all cases, the patients will prefer the alternative of trying to save the testicles to that of removing them.

12

Bed-wetting

Bed-wetting is one of the earliest male problems. It may seem a trivial subject to adults who wish to understand how their organs work. But back when they were five years old, for 15 percent of men bed-wetting was just about their biggest problem. By ten years of age 5 percent of boys still wet their beds, and as many as 2 percent of boys continue to wet their beds into the teen years.

Imagine what can happen to the boy's self-image while waiting for this poorly understood phenomenon to abate. Most assuredly the boy's mother will take him to the doctor many times. Depending upon the doctor's particular point of view, he may pontificate on its cause and propose any number of treatments. Most of the treatments he will propose have no scientific basis, and many of them are potentially harmful.

Some very famous people were bed wetters in their teens. A recent television special told of a very popular television star, Michael Landon, who was a bed wetter until his teens. His mother did everything wrong, including abuse and scolding, to try to shame him out of wetting his bed. She told him that if he wet his bed she would hang his bedsheets out of the window after school so that all of the kids in the neighborhood could see, thinking that if she embarrassed him enough he would stop. But it didn't stop the bed-wetting. After leaving school he would run home as fast as he could so that he could pull the bedsheets in from his bedroom window before his friends saw them.

Bed-wetting is the most poorly understood male problem. It will cure itself in the vast majority of cases without a physician's intervention. But bed-wetting is not insignificant. It is exasperating for parents and child alike. Furthermore, if a man lives to a ripe old age, he will have to deal with it once again.

A Response to Stress

According to Dr. Spock's famous book on baby and child care, the great majority of bed-wetting cases are due to tension in the child's life. According to this view, there are difficult situations in the young boy's growth that make him want unconsciously to retreat back into babyhood. Often these tensions are extremely trivial, such as moving into a new neighborhood. There is no point in scolding the boy. He usually feels bad enough about it himself. Children do not intentionally wet their beds. They do not intentionally want to aggravate their parents. It just automatically happens when they are asleep, perhaps in a dream reliving the distressing situation that is bothering them.

Many times the parents are so anxious to avoid this wet bed that they will get the child up at night, walk him over to the bathroom, and make him urinate in his sleep so that he will have an empty bladder for the rest of the night. Though this pragmatic approach clearly helps to keep the bed dry, Spock warns that doing this may just remind the boy that he is a baby and aggravate the basic cause of his bed-wetting. What he needs is to develop greater self-esteem and confidence that indeed he is not a baby.

Bed-wetting problems have been documented in history as far back as 1500 B.C., so we know it is not just a problem stemming from the pressures of modern life. The causes of bed-wetting were as prevalent 3,500 years ago as they are today.

In every phase of growing up, the little boy faces new landmarks of achievement that must be passed before he can continue his growth. If he cannot learn how to keep his pants and his bed dry, he will not feel very confident in tackling other problems, such as climbing the jungle gym, taking his first solo on a two-wheel bicycle, and even completing his lessons at school. Each failure aggravates the bed-wetting further by reinforcing his sense of inadequacy and failure. According to Spock, the little boy needs confidence and support from an adult he respects.

The problem will not be overcome in one night with the prescription of a pill, a night alarm, or an operation. Yet despite the simplicity and appeal of Spock's advice, most bed-wetting children today are subjected to a series of pseudosophisticated tests, treatments, and often surgery. Let's look at what modern medicine has brought to bear on this ancient problem.

The Urological Disease Approach

Most urologists recognize that bed-wetting is not usually a sign of any underlying bladder or kidney disease. Still, many urologists are not aware of this, and they may view bed-wetting as a subtle manifestation of a "serious urological condition" that could result in severe kidney damage and irreparable harm if not fully investigated with an armamentarium of telescopes, probes, X rays, and other diagnostic procedures that can be frightening if not damaging. Some doctors will schedule all of these tests on anyone with a urinary problem. Furthermore, the interpretation of some of these tests is very subjective.

Because of such mistaken views, some children with innocent variations in internal anatomy, which have nothing whatsoever to do with their bed-wetting, have been subjected to all varieties of surgery. One procedure (called meatotomy) often causes a urinary stream that goes in two directions (the so-called forked stream). Other children have gone through more serious operations, such as reimplantation of the ureter (the tube that conveys urine from the kidney into the bladder) or even removal of cysts from the prostate area. The latter operation can make the child permanently impotent, and the former can sometimes result in the loss of a kidney.

At the hands of some doctors, all boys who wet their beds will undergo cystoscopy. This means that a little telescope is inserted up the boy's penis into the bladder. Supposedly by viewing the inside of the bladder the urologist can learn something about any subtle disease process the child might have that could account for his bed-wetting.

The ironic thing about all these operations and procedures, whether "diagnostic" or "therapeutic," is that they frequently do cure the bed-wetting. Any child subjected to that sort of physical abuse and pain, because he is wetting his bed, is going to stop wetting his bed fairly soon. So if parents, frustrated with this seemingly insoluble problem, take the child to one of those urologists who believes that bed-wetting must be a sign of an underlying urologic abnormality, and if he subjects the child to any one of the combinations of the tortures just described, the bed-wetting may very well cease. But the possible complications of such totally irrational treatment are frightening. Ninety-nine percent of children who suffer from bed-wetting have no underlying urological disease.

The various tests that may be automatically and thoughtlessly used on a little boy are as follows.

In cystoscopy, a telescope is actually inserted up through the penis all the way into the bladder so that the doctor can view the inside of the bladder. This in itself is understandably terrifying to the child. But a bigger problem is that the urologist very frequently will see folds and wrinkles that are variations of the normal, but that could be interpreted as some sort of structural defect. He may even be tempted actually to operate on such wrinkles. The impression of objectivity in science can be awesome when it hides the subjectivity of the doctor.

Another test that some enthusiasts say is a must for children with bed-wetting is the so-called voiding cystourethrogram. With this test a rubber tube called a catheter is inserted through the child's penis, and his bladder is filled with a liquid which can be seen on X-ray. The liquid is fed slowly into the bladder until the child is miserably in pain and states that he can't hold his urine any longer. The catheter is then pulled out, and the child is told to urinate while X-ray pictures are taken. If some of the fluid leaks back toward the kidney, this reflux may tempt some surgeons to operate. The theory here is that reflux could ultimately damage the kidneys if left alone as the child grows up. Reflux itself has nothing to do with the child's bed-wetting problem, but many well-meaning urologists would be fearful that to leave the reflux undisturbed might potentially lead to kidney damage.

Another common test, called urodynamic testing, is designed to show whether the bed wetter's bladder reflexes have not matured. In an infant who has not yet been toilet trained, urination is by reflex. As he grows up, matures, and becomes toilet trained, he develops an automatic ability for his brain to control these reflexes and prevent the bladder from emptying involuntarily. But these tests have not demonstrated any abnormalities in bed wetters different from non-bed wetters. Yet this kind of testing became the rage in the late 1970s, and continues to be used in the fervent hope that some subtle abnormalities might be detected.

It used to be postulated that bed wetters sleep more deeply than non-bed wetters, and that this is the reason they have uncontrolled reflex bladder contractions in their sleep. But careful brain-wave sleep studies show that bed-wetting can occur in any phase of sleep, deep or light. Furthermore, bed wetters do not sleep any more deeply than non-bed wetters.

Thus, despite medical science's intensive and painful effort to find something wrong with bed wetters, it appears that bed-wetting is in fact a normal event. It begins at birth and is outgrown only because of social demand. Bed-wetting as a baby is considered normal. It is only for social reasons and convenience that it is not normal as one grows up.

Drug Therapy

If parents take their little bed-wetting boy to the doctor, it is probable he will eventually place the child on a drug called Tofranil. No one knows why or how this drug works to control bed-wetting, but most urologists seem to feel that it does improve the situation and decrease the number of wet nights. The major action of this drug is to pep up the brain and to cure mental depression. It is classified as a so-called "mood elevater." In mentally depressed adults this drug often cures their depression and increases their energy level. No one knows why it should have a positive effect on bed-wetting in little boys, but there are a number of popular theories about it.

One theory is that taking this drug before going to sleep will pep the youngster up sufficiently so that he will not be able to sleep very deeply. If the child is not sleeping deeply, then perhaps when his bladder fills with urine in the middle of the night he will feel the sensation of having to urinate, and will wake up and go to the bathroom without wetting his bed.

Another theory is that a side effect of this drug is to block the bladder reflexes. Such a blocking effect would not stop one from voluntarily and normally urinating, but it would prevent reflex contractions of the bladder. From the first day of a child's life, as his bladder fills with a small amount of urine, it automatically contracts once a certain level of distention has been reached. This is truly a reflex reaction, much like the leg jumping when the doctor taps the knee during a physical examination. The message does not travel to the brain and tell the infant it is time to urinate. The process happens automatically without the brain's intervention. Theoretically, if this drug Tofranil could block that automatic reaction, it could prevent bed-wetting. The problem with this theory is that drugs that are even more specifically designed to block this automatic reflex than Tofranil do not stop bed-wetting.

A third theory is that Tofranil actually causes the bladder's sphincter to tighten so much that even though the child's bladder may want to empty in the middle of the night, it cannot do so because the outlet of the bladder is held tight. A fourth theory is that if the child has some sort of psychological stress that is causing him to revert unconsciously to infancy, perhaps this mood-elevating drug artificially makes him feel a little better about himself. Since he goes to sleep feeling that much happier, perhaps he is less likely to wet his bed that night.

It should be obvious now that doctors really have no idea why this drug, which is handed out almost like popcorn to bed-wetting children, should be working. But a more important question is whether the drug itself is really improving the bed-wetting or whether it just has a placebo effect. In fact, giving the child a sugar pill is also extremely effective in reducing the number of wet nights. In the majority of studies comparing the effect of Tofranil to the effect of sugar pills in improving bed-wetting, Tofranil scored a little bit better than sugar pills, but sugar pills were dramatically more effective than doing nothing.

As early as 1968, forty separate studies had been reported around the world on the use of Tofranil for bed-wetting. Twenty-three of these studies were uncontrolled, which means the child was simply given the drug to see whether the bed-wetting nights were decreased, but were not compared to any group of children given sugar pills, or even to any group of children that were left untreated. Thus, any improvement that the child had after being given Tofranil could very easily have been from a purely psychological effect, or simply from a natural resolution of the problem, which frequently occurs with no treatment at all.

That left only seventeen studies that could be called controlled. Of those seventeen studies, eleven showed that Tofranil was effective, and six showed that it had no effect whatsoever. Thus by a simple majority ruling (rather than a clear-cut repeatable scientific observation), many clinicians assume that Tofranil should be used for little boys who wet their bed. It seems more likely that the design of some of these studies and the quality and accuracy of the reporting were highly variable. Because of the profound effects of the mind on this whole problem of bed-wetting, it is very hard to design a study that really demonstrates whether a particular drug is effective or not.

It is interesting to note that these drugs were rarely claimed to "cure" bed-wetting. The only alleged beneficial effect was to "improve" it. In other words, in a typical study the child might have had twenty wet nights per month before treatment, and fourteen wet nights per month after treatment. The researchers then say that this reduction in the number of wet nights by six per month is a "statistically significant" improvement, and feel that in some way this treatment is having a major effect. Any parent could tell these doctors that such an improvement isn't very significant. The numbers may impress the doctor theoretically on his charts, but they do not in any way reflect a "solution" to the problem. Thus, it appears that these drugs are not an answer to bed-wetting after all.

Furthermore, all drugs have side effects. Some children can become irritable and restless on Tofranil. Having it around the house creates a great risk of accidental overdosage. There have even been some fatal results when children unknowledgeably ingested over ten of these tablets at a time. To subject bed-wetting children to such potentially toxic medication is like blowing up the Golden Gate Bridge to get rid of a traffic jam. The only real advantage of drug treatment for bed-wetting is that it is terribly convenient simply to dispense a pill rather than to try to understand what is really happening inside the child and causing him to wet his bed.

Conditioning Therapy (Biofeedback)

Conditioning therapy is the most effective and rapid method of curing bed-wetting. Those who practice this therapy make no effort to understand the child's deeper thought processes or emotional stresses, but take the view that the bed-wetting is a practical problem that can be solved by training, and that success in the therapy will then give the child a better self-image. It is a very pragmatic approach, which comes out of the whole school of behaviorism in psychology. According to this view, the stresses that cause the child to wet his bed in the first place are probably not as great as the stress created by the fact that he is bed-wetting. Thus if the therapist neglects the basic underlying psychological problem that is causing the bed-wetting, and solves the behavioral abnormality itself, the child's view of himself will improve, and he will be better able to cope with the other stresses in his life.

The great Russian psychologist Pavlov first demonstrated at the turn of the century that if you rang a bell whenever you brought food to a hungry dog, eventually ringing the bell alone would make the dog's mouth salivate. The dog has been "conditioned" to salivate in response to the ringing of a bell. Now in the 1980s this basic concept has blossomed into one of the most rapidly growing fields of psychotherapy, biofeedback.

Biofeedback has been used to condition people out of all sorts of undesirable behavior patterns, such as stuttering, sleep-walking, and even improper tennis strokes and smoking. There is a very practical appeal to this approach. For example, if a child is stuttering at two and a half years of age, should he be taken to an ear, nose, and throat doctor to find out if he has some kind of physical problem causing him to stutter, or should he perhaps be taken to a speech therapist who will use training methods to condition him out of his stuttering? If the child's stuttering is caused by a basic insecurity, perhaps related to moving to a new community or the arrival of a new sibling, would it be better to deal with his basic underlying insecurity, or to try to train him out of it with biofeedback?

The basic tenet of conditioning therapy is that psychological disturbances are best understood as being the result of either a failure to learn or the acquisition of poorly adapted patterns of behavior. In the case of bed-wetting, the behavior therapist argues that the child has failed to acquire a conditioned response of arousal at a point when the bladder is filled. The aim of treatment is to provide the patient with a chance to learn what he has not learned yet in his normal course of maturation. In contrast, in the traditional psychiatric approach, where bed-wetting is interpreted as a signal of an underlying psychological disturbance, the symptom of bed-wetting is not even treated. Instead, the psychiatrist tries to treat the underlying psychological disturbance and hopes the bed-wetting will automatically disappear. The behavior therapist feels that this will take too much time and would probably not work in many cases anyway. He therefore goes straight to the symptom of bed-wetting, and tries to bypass any effort at insight.

There are two ways of conditioning a child not to wet his bed. One utilizes an alarm wake-up device. This device can be purchased from a company called Palco in San Francisco, or Nytone Alarm Company in Salt Lake City, for about thirty-five dollars. A little portable alarm is worn on the child's wrist and connected to sensors in his pajamas that will make the alarm go off if he urinates in his pajamas and gets them wet. The alarm wakes the child up just as he is beginning to urinate so that he then knows to get out of bed and complete the act of urination in the toilet. After a week of this conditioning, the child begins to wake up spontaneously just before he would normally wet his bed, and goes to the toilet instead. There will be frequent relapses of bed-wetting at first, but eventually 80 percent of such children will essentially have been trained out of their bed-wetting after about a month.

Some of the older devices for this purpose were electronically very poor and either woke the child too late, or in fact never woke him at all, but did manage to wake the rest of the family. The bed wetter frequently slept through the pandemonium. So this therapy did not work very well before the recent development of more sophisticated electronics.

The view that curing the bed-wetting without approaching the basic psychological cause would cause other psychological problems simply has not turned out to be true. A child feels so much better about himself after having been trained out of bed-wetting that, if anything, he is better able to deal with the stresses within his family.

But conditioning therapy does not have to rely on an electronic urine-activated alarm system. A urologist colleague of mine, who is a very athletic, "macho" person, recently admitted to me that he was a bed wetter until the age of twelve. He has a great deal of insight into this problem and seems to know more about it than any other urologist or parent I know. He understood his own psychodynamics and could actually explain to me what was going on inside his head as he was wetting his bed, and how he overcame it. His approach to boys with this problem seems to use the best of conditioning therapy and yet allows the parents and everyone involved to understand the stresses that help to cause the bed-wetting in the first place.

He relates that as a child sleeping at night, just about to wet his bed, he was in a sort of a twilight awareness of what was about to happen, and knew that if he woke up he would be able to get out of bed and make it to the bathroom. But he really didn't want to wake up. It was so comfortable and so cozy in that bed that when it came right down to it at that particular moment he couldn't see giving up the comfort and security of that nice bed and that comfortable sleep just to get up and empty his bladder. So he actually urinated in his bed while allowing himself to continue to sleep. It was occurring somewhere between consciousness and unconsciousness, and he wasn't really aware of the dynamics of what was going on inside his head until he became somewhat older, around the age of twelve.

A variety of stresses in a little boy's life can cause him to wet his bed in this way. He simply finds it more comfortable to retain the security of being asleep. Even though in the morning he regrets the wet bed, feels ashamed of himself, and wishes he had not done it, nonetheless he is unable to get out of this habit easily.

This urologist's approach to his patients is very similar to the alarm system of conditioning I mentioned earlier. But he doesn't use fancy mechanical or electronic devices. He simply gives the parents the following instructions. Make sure the child goes to bed early, at eight o'clock or so. The parents should then wake the child at eleven P.M. or midnight. Usually this is before the child will have wet his bed. It will not be easy to wake the child, but they must make sure to wake him with a great deal of love and attention. They should not wake him in a punitive way and should not be angry because he doesn't wake up immediately. They should just get him out of bed and wake him up with an arm around him, giving him all of the warmth and security he needs. Once they are certain that he is awake, they give him a number to remember that he can recite back to them the next morning, and give him a reward the next morning for remembering that number. This ensures that he will recollect the fact that he did get up at night.

Then they take him to the bathroom and allow him to urinate, after which they return him to his bed and let him go to sleep again. Then they set their alarm for three or four A.M., wake themselves up, go to his bed, and wake him up one more time in the same way that they did the first time. They should then repeat the entire process, giving him a new number to remember this time. Then the parents can return to bed and reset their alarm for normal wake-up time.

With this approach to conditioning, just like with the alarm system, the child will eventually learn to get up on his own when he feels the urge to urinate. Eventually, after many months he will learn subconsciously to control the need to urinate while he is asleep, and may not even get up in the middle of the night anymore.

Both of these approaches to conditioning, or behavior modification therapy, work extremely well in over 80 percent of boys. It always seems so much easier just to prescribe a pill like Tofranil. But the pill simply doesn't work much better than a placebo, relapses in bed-wetting are the rule, and the pill can have some very disconcerting if not dangerous side effects, such as restlessness, tearfulness, and difficulty with concentration, as well as insomnia and nervous irritability.

Most of the physicians that the boy may see with his parents will be unfamiliar with the pragmatic behavior-modification approach. They may perform thousands of dollars' worth of tests and then either place him on drug therapy or refer him to a psychiatrist.

Sometimes the parents have better common sense and understand the problem better than the doctor. I recently saw a seven-and-a-half-year-old boy whose older brother was toilet trained at three years with great difficulty, but once trained never wet his bed. But this little boy was a problem bed wetter. He was extremely bright, ahead of the other kids in his class, a good athlete, and had many friends. But he performed poorly in school despite testing several grades ahead of himself simply because of boredom with classroom routine that was below his intellectual level. He had been bed-wetting for over four years, so his mother finally tired of all the doctor's platitudes, and purchased one of the buzzer alarm systems. Within one week the child was dry at night for the first time in four years. By the time she saw me she had discontinued the alarm device, and the child's bed remained dry. The only reason she even consulted me was to find out if she had done something wrong. What she did, in fact, was to awaken me to the benefits of a pragmatic approach to a problem that has been totally overintellectualized both psychodynamically and pharmaceutically.

Psychotherapy

A common criticism of these practical conditioning techniques for curing bed-wetting is that they deal only with the symptoms and do not help the patient to achieve insight into the underlying conflicts that are presumed to be the cause of his problem. A fear many psychiatrists have is that by curing or removing such bad habits, of which bed-wetting is only one example, without curing the basic underlying cause, such as tension in the environment or internal psychological conflict, other symptoms of the basic stress will appear to replace the one that has been conditioned away. This criticism from psychiatrists applies not only to bed-wetting, but also to stuttering, ticks, and even bad habits such as smoking, drinking, and thumb-sucking.

This view has been challenged by modern behavior therapists, who regard a symptom such as bed-wetting as simply an undesirable habit and a response acquired historically through a faulty learning experience of the child. These symptoms or habits can be eliminated in the most direct manner simply by conditioning. They are merely maladapted anxiety responses that must be snuffed out directly. Thus, the neurotic responses of bed-wetting, thumb-sucking, stuttering, a tick, or even smoking, drinking, or gambling are not seen as mechanisms for avoiding conflict or stress but rather as harmful stress responses in themselves.

It is therefore often necessary to shape or condition new motor habits by whatever behavioral technique is pragmatically most appropriate. Bed-wetting is admittedly just a symptom of underlying stress, but according to the behavior therapist, these symptoms are not helpful responses to the stress. By eliminating these maladapted and unhelpful symptoms, the child will find it easier to deal with whatever stress does still exist in his environment.

The psychoanalyst's argument that new symptoms will develop out of the suppression of old symptoms has now been largely disproved. Children who are conditioned pragmatically and taught not to wet their bed, despite the original stress that may have caused their bed-wetting in the first place, do not seem to develop new maladaptive symptoms. Thus, the fear that symptom substitution would attend this relatively superficial and pragmatic approach to the child's problem simply is not borne out. Furthermore, behaviorists argue that very often by the time the psychiatrist or psychoanalyst has seen the bed-wetting child, the stress that precipitated the bed-wetting may be gone from his life. Yet he has been conditioned in this maladaptive way already to wet his bed. In other words, he has acquired a bad habit. This bad habit will not automatically go away simply because the patient is made aware of the underlying stress that originally precipitated it. This bad habit must be conditioned away just as it was originally conditioned in.

Summary

Bed-wetting is one of the earliest and most trying male problems. It can lead to terrible embarrassment and loss of confidence. To compound this problem the child may be seen by a doctor who will insert a telescope up his penis, possibly cut out a section of his sphincter, certainly perform many X rays, maybe place him on a drug that will make him restless, irritable, and unable to sleep, or simply tell him not to worry about it because he will grow out of it. Even such barbaric treatments as using a clamp on the penis and drugs to prevent urination altogether have been tried occasionally in an attempt to deal in a simple fashion with what after all appears to be nothing more than a very bad habit resulting from stress of one kind or another.

These children are not deliberately wetting their beds. They are not doing this to get even with their parents, and in turn their parents should not be trying to get even with them. There is no need to scold or shame the boy for bed-wetting, because he usually feels bad enough about it himself. He should not be made to hang out his sheets so that other boys will learn of his disgrace. He wants to be dry at night but does not seem to have any control over the unconscious reflex wetting that occurs in the middle of his sleep.

Dr. Spock's basic approach is one of simple encouragement, giving the child confidence that soon he will be a man and will grow out of this problem. It is as though he is suggesting that simply by removing or correcting the stress in the child's life, bed-wetting will automatically go away. Yet we know that the bed-wetting in itself is not a helpful response to the child's problem. Furthermore, sometimes successfully removing from his environment the stress that helped to precipitate the bed-wettting will not necessarily do away with this bad habit that he has now formed.

Certainly time, encouragement, sympathy, and perhaps even psychotherapy to help the child deal with his conflicts will eventually result in the cure of his bed-wetting problem. But a practical behavior modification approach is now gaining increasing popularity in the United States because of its high cure rate, and may be the best common sense solution of all. Many doctors say simply to do nothing and regard bed-wetting as a natural event in growing up and point out that 98 percent of boys will have spontaneously been cured by the age of fifteen without treatment at all. But all of the young men in their early teens I have talked to who are still afflicted with bed-wetting, with all of its crushing embarrassment and tension, would have been quite happy to have been conditioned out of this bad habit of theirs at a much earlier age.

13

Is It a Boy?

At the beginning of our lives we are all one common undifferentiated sex. For the first forty days of an embryo's development, the structures that in boys will turn into male organs are absolutely the same as those that in girls will become female organs. However, if the embryo is to become a boy, testicles develop at forty days after conception, and these testicles direct the development of all the other male organs. A female ovary, on the other hand, is not necessary to mastermind or direct the embryo's development into a female. If testicles do not develop at this critical time, it will be born a female. Even if there is no ovary whatsoever, the normal embryological development of the human in the absence of testicles is toward becoming a structural female. If a male embryo were castrated at forty days' development, it would not grow up neutrally. It would become a female. The development into a female is simply the normal course of human events.

When something goes wrong in the restructuring of the genitals of a child that is genetically male, it may not make it quite all the way out of the female mold. The male genital development is then "unfinished," and the infant may be born with what doctors call "ambiguous genitalia." Understanding how our male organs develop, how they may not have developed completely, and seeing the similarity between each male genital structure and its female counterpart will help all men to understand their sexual identity better.

The Internal Sex Organs

Before six weeks of development inside the mother's womb, males and females look exactly the same. But the female embryo has XX chromosomes in every cell of her developing body that will eventually program her into becoming a female, and the male embryo has XY chromosomes that will program him into becom-

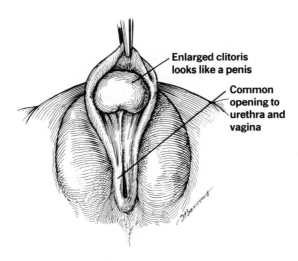

Enlarged clitoris looks like a penis

Common opening to urethra and vagina

Ambiguous Genitalia

ing a boy. Both boys and girls at this age have primitive gonads, which in the girl will soon become ovaries and in the boy likewise become testicles. It is not until the primitive gonad differentiates specifically into testicles that the male genital structures will thereafter begin to develop.

At six weeks of development the testicles have just begun to form, making the tubules that will ultimately create sperm and the cells that will make male hormone. In females the ovary does not form this soon. Females continue to have an undifferentiated gonad for another three months. Thus the female's development occurs under no specific guidance or control. It is simply the natural unfolding of events.

It is the Y chromosome in the male child that causes his primitive gonad to become a testicle. If the Y chromosome is not successful in causing the development of testicles, then none of the other male structures will develop either. The Y chromosome does not automatically make the embryo male; it simply creates testicles, and it is the testicle that then causes the embryo to become male. If anything goes wrong with the testicles, the fetus may not become a boy even though its XY genes say that it should be.

The ovaries, the Fallopian tubes, and the uterus (i.e., the womb) are the female's internal sex organs. The male's internal sex organs are the prostate gland, the seminal vesicles, which provide the fluid that carries the sperm, the vas deferens (sperm duct), the testicles, and the epididymis. During the early, neutral period of sexual development, there are two basic duct systems that will develop into these male or female internal sex organs. These are called the Wolffian and Müllerian ducts. These ducts function as kidneys in the early phase of our development as embryos. They are no longer needed because later in embryonic life we develop a much more refined kidney system. These two primitive kidneys are what form the internal sex organs of men and women.

In the female embryo, the Wolffian duct degenerates because there is no male hormone (testosterone) to sustain it, but the Müllerian duct develops into the Fallopian tubes, uterus, and

even the upper third of the vagina. In the male embryo the opposite occurs. The Müllerian duct degenerates under the guidance
of the testicles, but the Wolffian duct develops fully into the vas
deferens, epididymis, seminal vesicles, and ejaculatory duct.

All men have located near their prostate gland at the base
of their ejaculatory duct a little uterus and a little vagina which
are remnants of the Müllerian duct. This embryonic vagina is

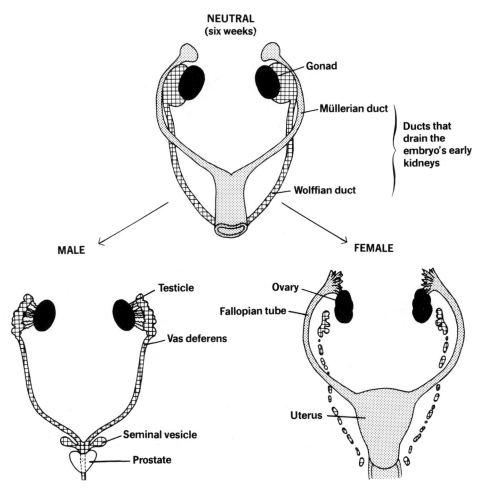

Formation of Male and Female Internal Sex Organs

called the verumontanum, or the prostatic utricle. Every time a urologist looks inside the penis at the prostate gland (a relatively common diagnostic procedure called cystoscopy), he can see this vestigial vagina, which is a permanent testament to our origins as one common sex. In the same fashion, every woman has an embryonic prostate gland that never fully develops, since the prostate gland in the male forms from the same little glands that also surround the opening to the female bladder.

To summarize, the testicles direct the female internal structures to degenerate and the male internal structures to grow and develop. Each testicle molds the development of its particular side. Thus if we had a testicle on one side of the little embryo and an ovary on the other side (or no testicle at all on the other side), the Müllerian duct would not regress, the Wolffian duct would not grow, and on the side without a testicle the child would have all the internal reproductive structures of a female, including Fallopian tube, uterus, and even the upper portion of a vagina. But most men with only one testicle are normal males and have no uterus, tubes, or vagina, indicating that they had both testicles when they were embryos, but that one of the testicles degenerated before birth.

The External Sex Organs

Although men and women appear superficially to be markedly different in the appearance of their external genitals, a closer look will demonstrate just how similar the sexes actually are. All of the external sex organs—the labia, vagina, and clitoris in the female and the penis and scrotal sac in the male—develop from the same embryologic structures. The male penis is essentially no different from the female clitoris, except that it is bigger. The male scrotum is no different from the female's labia majora except that it is larger and contains testicles.

Before the little embryo finds out whether it is a boy or a girl, its external sex organs consist of the genital tubercle (this becomes the penis in a boy and the clitoris in a girl), the genital swellings (these become the labia majora in a female and the scrotum in a male), and the urethral fold or grooves (this becomes the labia minora of the vagina in a female and the penile urethra in a male). Without the hormone testosterone produced by the embryo's own testicles, the natural tendency is for these external genitalia to become female. It is only the presence of a testicle that imposes upon the embryo's otherwise natural inclination toward becoming a female, the structures of the male external genitalia instead.

The male's penis and scrotum develop in the womb before he is three months old. The genital tubercle lengthens into a true penis so that it no longer looks like a clitoris, and the penile urethral folds elongate and fuse, allowing the little boy to urinate out of the tip. Between seven months of embryonic life and just shortly before birth the testicles begin their descent from the abdomen into the scrotum.

The descent of the testicles is a remarkable event. During most of fetal life, and long after the penis and scrotum have been properly sculpted, the testicles remain within the abdomen, where the ovaries reside in the female. In fact, inside the abdomen they look superficially just like ovaries, are in the same position, and are supported by the same ligaments that support the ovaries. Then at about seven months they literally push their way through the peritoneum (the envelope containing all of the abdominal organs) down into the scrotum. If they create too big an opening which fails to seal, a hernia results. Later, when a man lifts and strains heavily, putting stress on his hernia, he is squeezing the abdominal contents out through this same little hole, which was left after his testicles first descended.

The foreskin develops equally in males and females, and testosterone has no effect in stimulating or enhancing its growth. In the female the foreskin obscures the clitoris. In the male the penis is so large that the foreskin is a more prominent structure. But the foreskin is the only genital organ which, after all of its embryonic development, is essentially the same in men and women.

Formation of Male and Female External Sex Organs

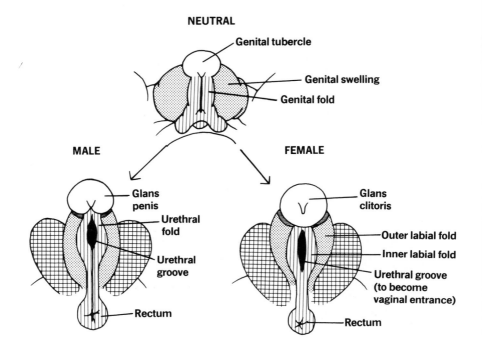

NEUTRAL

Genital tubercle

Genital swelling

Genital fold

MALE

Glans penis

Urethral fold

Urethral groove

Rectum

FEMALE

Glans clitoris

Outer labial fold

Inner labial fold

Urethral groove (to become vaginal entrance)

Rectum

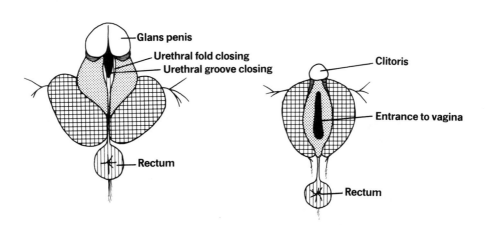

Glans penis

Urethral fold closing

Urethral groove closing

Rectum

Clitoris

Entrance to vagina

Rectum

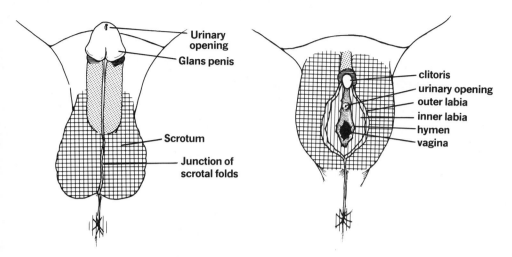

Errors in the Baby's Sex

One of the first questions every new parent is anxiously awaiting the answer to as soon as the baby is pushed out of the womb is whether it is a boy or a girl. The doctor's answer to that question is based on a very quick glance at the genital area. In most cases, it is easy to give an immediate answer. But sometimes the genitalia are a bit confusing, and it is not really clear whether it is a boy or a girl.

Nature's plan for the developing embryo during its nine months in the womb is to take the same initial structures and gradually modify them into either male or female genitals. The genital tubercle grows into a penis in males or retracts and curves underneath to become a clitoris in females. In a boy, folds of skin literally wrap around the penis and join on the underside to form the urethral canal through which he urinates, while in a girl it opens into the labia minora. What becomes the scrotal skin in the male, meeting in the midline and fusing, becomes the labia majora, the so-called portals to the vagina in the female. If this relatively simple plan of biologic engineering is not completed, then the baby will look neither fully male nor fully female. The baby can be born in literally an unfinished state of sexual development and it can be very difficult to tell by a glance whether it is a boy or a girl. A large clitoris is not very much different from a small penis.

If the opening from which the little boy urinates is located near the scrotal area instead of coming out from the tip of the penis, and if his penis is retracted downward toward this area, it doesn't look very much different from a clitoris. If a girl's vagina is partially fused at the opening, it may be so small that it really looks like the urinary meatus of a little boy whose penis didn't develop properly. But if a doctor puts a telescope through this little meatus he may be surprised to find that instead of looking into the bladder he is instead looking into the vagina of what after all is a little girl with a larger than normal clitoris. If a baby comes out with this unfinished external sexual development, the parents will be thoroughly confused as to what sex he or she is.

SEVEN WEEK OLD MALE EMBRYO **NINE WEEK OLD MALE EMBRYO**

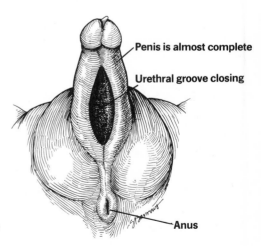

Genital tubercle

Urogenital fold

Would become entrance to vagina if this were to become a girl

Penis is almost complete

Urethral groove closing

Anus

Formation of the Penis in the Womb

Most of these babies with ambiguous genitalia (see page 143) are either boys or girls genetically, although their sexual development is confusing and unclear. In some cases, they are truly neither boys nor girls but hermaphrodites, which means that they have both a testicle and an ovary. "Hermaphrodite" is an early Greek word that means half boy and half girl. The testicle on one side directs development of male sex organs, while an ovary or the absence of a testicle on the other side allows the development of female sex organs.

Usually the child with ambiguous genitalia is not a true hermaphrodite, but is either a boy or a girl. It has either ovaries or testicles, but for some reason the process of developing the sex organs failed during fetal life. We call these more common cases "pseudohermaphrodites" or "false hermaphrodites." They are either boys or girls but they don't look like either.

The most common type of false hermaphrodite is the female false hermaphrodite. This is an otherwise normal female with a uterus, vagina, Fallopian tubes, and ovaries. The problem is that too much male hormone was produced while she was undergoing fetal development. This male hormone caused her clitoris to grow large, so it looks like a penis, and her vagina to close up

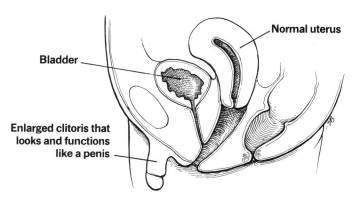

Female False Hermaphrodite (side view)

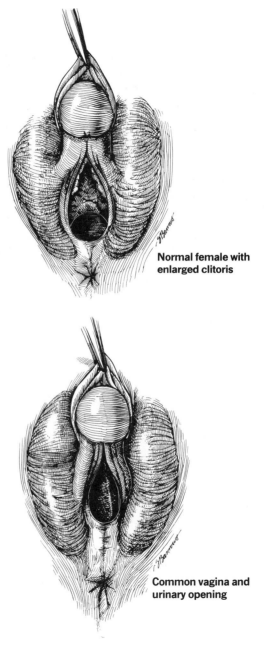

**Normal female with
enlarged clitoris**

**Common vagina and
urinary opening**

Four Degrees of Male Appearance in Female False Hermaphrodites

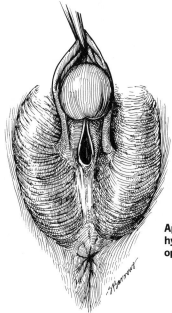

**Appears to be male with
hypospadias urinary
opening**

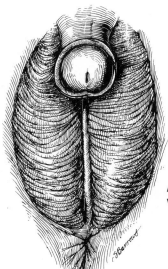

**Appears to be male
with undescended testicles**

partly, so it resembles the urinary meatus. She doesn't look like a boy in most cases because there are no testicles in the scrotum, and the penis, though much larger than a normal clitoris, is usually bent over and rather small. If the baby's genes are examined through relatively simple blood tests, it is found to be a normal XX female, but she simply has too much male hormone. In some severe cases, a female false hermaphrodite will look exactly like a boy with undescended testicles and a normal penis urinating out of the tip. There have been a few of these girls (with normal vaginas, uterus, Fallopian tubes, and ovaries hidden inside) who have been raised completely as boys only to discover in their late teens, after careful medical evaluation, that they are in fact girls.

These female false hermaphrodites are fairly common. They are caused by a defect in the adrenal gland whereby the gland makes more male hormone than it is supposed to make. Fortunately, if the diagnosis is made properly, these little girls can be placed on cortisone tablets, which suppress the adrenal's production of the inappropriately large amount of male hormone. Occasionally the same problem can be caused by the mother taking certain hormones during her pregnancy. Whatever the origin of the excess of male hormone, it causes the girl fetus to come out looking partly like a boy. Fortunately, it can be treated simply. Surgery can open up the sealed-off vagina and reduce the size of the penis so that it looks more like a proper clitoris. These babies should grow up to be normal, happy, healthy girls, if the diagnosis is made early enough so that they are not raised as boys.

Male false hermaphrodites are somewhat less common than female false hermaphrodites. A male false hermaphrodite has two normal testicles and genetically he is a normal XY boy, but he is born looking just like a girl. The testicles are undescended, the penis resembles a small clitoris, and there is a normal vagina (somewhat shortened), but no uterus, no ovaries, and no Fallopian tubes. These boys look just exactly like females. The only doubt as to their complete femininity is the presence of two lumps in the groin area of the abdomen which in truth are testicles. Otherwise there is no reason to suspect that those babies are anything but normal girls. Yet they are genetically male, with normal testicles and no female internal genitalia. Such children may not ever find out that they are boys.

The cause of this problem in most cases is that for some reason all of the cells of the child's body are insensitive to the stimulatory effects of male hormone. The testicles are making a perfectly adequate amount of testosterone, which normally should mold the development of the genitals into those of a boy. But all of his cells are totally unresponsive to the hormone, and thus he develops neutrally, which as we know is always female.

Since his testicles are normal, they produce Müllerian inhibiting factor, which causes the Müllerian duct to degenerate rather than form into Fallopian tubes, uterus, and upper vagina. Unfortunately, therefore, this boy does not develop any female internal genitalia, but the external genitalia, which are only molded into male genitalia by testosterone, develop neutrally, which is female. Although a normal external vagina forms, it is not very deep because the deepest recesses of the vagina develop out of the same Müllerian duct from which the uterus develops. Surgery is necessary to deepen the vagina in these "girls" in order to allow adequate intercourse with a male partner.

The usual treatment for such a "male" false hermaphrodite is to remove the testicles from the abdomen at puberty, and to simply raise the child as a normal girl. Such individuals usually grow and function very well as girls and develop a completely feminine psychosexual identity. But hidden in all of the cells throughout her body are XY chromosomes, indicating that long ago she was originally destined to be a boy.

The only unsolvable problem with these "girls" is that they don't ever grow pubic hair. In boys as well as girls, pubic hair and hair under the arms will grow only in response to the male hormone, testosterone. All girls produce some testosterone, though in much smaller amounts than boys. But no amount of male hormone, or for that matter female hormone, and no treatment known to man can make these "girls" ever grow pubic hair.

The major disaster in this syndrome occurs when one of these male false hermaphrodites has only a partial insensitivity to testosterone, and has a sufficiently large penis with a properly fused vagina that he looks enough like a boy that a decision is made to raise him as a boy. When he reaches puberty, however, he develops feminine breasts and does not develop normal masculine body traits since his body is still resistant to male sex hormone. His voice remains high-pitched, his face unbearded, and his body feminine rather than masculine in contour. His body is unresponsive to the normal increase in male hormone at puberty. Thus he remains a totally inadequate male because of a mistaken decision at birth to raise him as a boy, simply because his external genitalia were not completely female and because he had male genes. He would have been far better off undergoing surgery as a child to reduce the size of his penis to that of a clitoris and to create a vagina.

Tragedies like this are not uncommon in our everyday life. False hermaphrodites are common but not often talked about. Recently I read in the newspaper that Stella Walsh, the famous woman Olympic star of the 1930s who broke all records in track and won five gold medals as well as three silver medals, one bronze medal, and sixty-five world records, was shot and killed during a robbery at a department store, and this required that an autopsy be performed. At the autopsy, to everyone's complete shock, it was discovered that she had an intersex problem that had never been talked about, and that in truth she was a genetic male. Apparently she was a wonderful woman who was not only a great athlete, but was loved by everyone. But she was never able to consummate a marital relationship and indeed stayed with her husband for only about six weeks. Certainly it would be unlikely that in those early days she had any kind of sex change surgery, but was rather certainly suffering from some sort of congenital hermaphroditic condition. Since she was raised as a girl, she developed a completely normal psychosocial female identity, but because of a genital abnormality, probably represented by an enlarged penislike clitoris and a small vagina, she was never able to consummate fully her identity as a woman. Both women and men with confusing sex characteristics (which we lump together under one term, ambiguous genitalia) abound in our society, but their condition is kept a secret because of shame and embarrassment. Yet diagnosis in infancy with proper medical and surgical treatment can spare these children the mental torture that this famous athletic star must have gone through for the sixty-nine years of her life.

In almost all cases of ambiguous genitalia, a pragmatic decision must be made as to whether to raise the child as a boy or a girl, based upon how easy it is to change his or her genitalia from neutral to either the male or the female side. Since it is usually easier to change toward the female, most children with this kind of an intersex problem are designated as females, with appropriate surgical correction in that direction, and they grow up with perfectly normal psychosexual identity as females. The sex of rearing, going back to the earliest months of life, is the most important factor in determining the child's identity as a boy or a girl. Their genetic sex (whether XY or XX), or even what kind of gonads they have (whether testicles or ovaries), are completely insignificant in determining their sexual identity. An arbitrary designation of male or female carried out from birth onward by the parents is what determines the child's psychosexual identity.

Ambiguous Genitalia in Otherwise Normal Boys

In most of the intersex cases, the sexual designation at birth ought to be female because it is so difficult surgically and hormonally to restructure an intersex child into a male. But the child with ambiguous genitalia may frequently be a normal male who simply has a penis deformity or undescended testicles. These boys can have relatively simple surgical reconstruction, and then grow up as fertile young men without any difficulty. These boys are not hermaphrodites, but are simply normal males whose external genitals did not quite finish their development by the time they were born, and surgical assistance is needed to complete the job. Congenital abnormalities of the male genitalia are the most common birth defects. They are not occasional freak cases. Boys with such conditions can and must have corrective surgery before the age of five.

The most common type of "unfinished penis" is called hypospadias. This is a condition in which there is an unfused open gutter on the underside of the penis instead of a closed urethral tube, and the child urinates from a little opening at the base of the penis near his scrotum instead of at the tip (see page 153). This type of penis usually has a severe curve to it, and when the child gets an erection it cannot straighten out like a normal penis. This bowing is called a chordee, and is a condition that comes in all degrees of severity. In its most severe state, the penis is bowed under so far into the scrotum that it literally looks like a large clitoris.

I recently corrected such a defect in a little boy whose mother was told shortly after his birth that he was neither a girl nor a boy but somewhere in between. This kind of confusing statement from an unknowledgeable doctor can create an ambiguity in the parent's thinking about the child that can destroy the child's psychosexual identity of rearing. Fortunately, this mother was smarter than the doctor, and went to a laboratory for genetic testing, which showed that the child was a normal XY boy. After several months his testicles came down into his scrotum and it was apparent that this boy was not a hermaphrodite. He was simply a normal little boy whose penis never quite finished its development. Surgery (which was not terribly complicated) completely corrected the unfinished state of his penis, and he is now a normal little boy, indistinguishable physically or psychologically from any other.

In all of these cases, the child's gender identity is not preordained or determined specifically by his genes or his gonads. Psychosexual identity as a boy, or as a girl results from the process of social stimulation and experience. It is important not to allow ambiguity of the genitalia to result in an ambiguity of rearing which can handicap the child throughout life, wondering exactly what or who he or she is.

PART FOUR
Gender Identity and Homosexuality

14

Clearing Up the Myths

Everyone in our society would like to know what it is that predisposes a man toward homosexuality, transsexualism, fetishism, or paraphilia. Is it genetically programmed? Does it develop in earliest childhood or in adolescence? Is it related to hormone output? These are terribly painful questions for parents who fear that exposure to homosexual behavior may cause previously heterosexual persons—their children or even their spouses—to become homosexuals.

But are such fears realistic? When is sexual preference established, and how? Can sexual preference change?

These questions open up a huge arena of controversy, but fortunately there is now factual information that provides answers to many of them. In answering these questions, we will first define the various behaviors that are often mistaken as homosexuality, and address the many common misconceptions about gender identity and sexual preference. Then we will discuss the stages of development of sexual identity in little boys. We will summarize the considerable body of evidence about how sexual identity develops in children with ambiguous genitalia, and how it is confused in children who grow up to be transsexuals. Using the solid

161

data now available in these extreme situations, we will then discuss the probable causes of homosexuality, which is much more common, and which we have finally come to understand better.

The Kinsey Report

Back in 1948, Alfred C. Kinsey's famous study of human sexual behavior made it clear that homosexuality is very common among men and relatively uncommon among women. According to Kinsey, many adult males have had at least one homosexual experience; only 3 to 4 percent maintain exclusively homosexual activity, however; and the male orgasms resulting from homosexual contact constitute only 6 percent of the total number of orgasms. Kinsey also observed that there is a large number of normal heterosexual men who, if the circumstances are right, might turn to a homosexual relationship. The best example of this behavior, known even in the 1940s, is the relationships that form between male prisoners confined for long periods of time.

It is not entirely clear why more males than females should choose homosexual behavior. One possible explanation is that the little girl has much greater opportunity to identify with her mother than the little boy has to model himself on his father, especially since the boy is totally dependent on his mother early in life.

Another reason for the greater occurrence of gender confusion in men than women is the male's greater dependence on *visual* erotic stimulation. The human male, unlike most animals, is attracted to the female primarily through visual cues. When the little boy begins to go through puberty, his first complete sexual experience is usually the so-called wet dream, in which he imagines having sex with a girl. The adolescent girl has no corresponding dream experience. A girl may, of course, respond to the sight of a good-looking boy, but not usually with the same intensity of physical excitement that a boy would have in seeing a good-looking girl. The female relies more on romantic interchange and touch for sexual stimulation, whereas the adolescent boy is strictly visual in his erotic arousal.

When most young boys begin to masturbate, they have visual fantasies in which they imagine having sexual relations with a girl. While some young boys may experience orgasm simply from viewing a woman they find attractive, most young girls require tactile stimulation to achieve such a level of excitation. This sensitivity to *visual* stimuli for sexual arousal may be related to the male's greater production of testosterone. This hormone is responsible in both boys and girls for sexual desire, and males have much more of it than females. Transsexualism and homosexuality may be related to a disorientation of the little boy's visual images of sexuality, which become firmly set at an early age, and to which a little girl is much less susceptible due to her lower testosterone levels.

Homosexuality, Transsexualism, Transvestism, Intersex, and Paraphilia

A great deal is known about transsexuals and about what causes their gender confusion. Although less is known about the homosexual, the transvestite, and the paraphiliac, these conditions probably stem from causes similar to the more extreme case of the transsexual. So let's define these terms.

A *homosexual* male is a man who has a clearly established male identity but who may not have a clearly established sexual preference. If his sexual preference is clearly identified, it is toward an individual of the same gender. A man who desires sex only with other men is called an obligatory homosexual, whereas a man who in some circumstances is willing to have sex with women, and in other circumstances with men, is called a facultative homosexual, or a bisexual.

A *transsexual* is a man who does not see himself as a man at all. He is without question a male genetically, hormonally, and structurally, but mentally he sees himself as a female trapped within a male's body. The male transsexual does not want to have sex with male homosexuals or with other male transsexuals. He literally despises his sex organs and longs to be rid of them and to have sex with normal heterosexual men. Interestingly, the more firmly rooted and secure the transsexual's female identity is, the less likely he is to have exaggerated effeminate mannerisms. Such transsexuals have *normal* female mannerisms, rather than the caricatures of female mannerisms that we think of as effeminate.

The *transvestite* alternates between male and female identity. The male transvestite is a man who wants to have sex with females, but who can do so successfully only while dressed as and pretending to be female. The rest of the time the transvestite behaves as a normal male. He does not want to change his sex to become a female. That is the desire of the transsexual. Furthermore, unlike the homosexual, he does not want to have sex with other men.

The transvestite suffers intolerable anxiety if he does not dress from time to time in female clothes. Transvestites may not discover their preference until puberty, when they wish to masturbate but find they can only achieve orgasm while wearing or holding some article of female clothing. Sometimes in later adulthood the transvestite decides to cross-dress as a female permanently, and in such cases may be very difficult to distinguish from a transsexual. But most transvestites spend all of their lives with two personalities, one female and one male. While male, the transvestite is usually masculine and domineering and while female, he is a model of femininity. The two sides of this individual's gender confusion have simply never melted together.

The borderline between the transvestite and the transsexual can be very confusing. After going through sex-change surgery, one so-called male transsexual is reported to have become a lesbian. She was happy to be a woman rather than a man, but still preferred sex with women. This case sounds almost like that of a transvestite—a male who prefers sex with women but has to think of himself as a woman while he is doing it.

Paraphilia is a form of gender confusion in which the man can only achieve erotic fulfillment when a specific image is achieved. The sex criminal who rapes children has a paraphilia in which he has an intense erotic need that can only be fulfilled by having forcible sex with a child. It is a specific type of sexual fixation in a particular man that must be fulfilled in order for him to have sexual gratification. Most psychologists feel that paraphilia develops when a child experiences punishment and guilt for the normal heterosexual expressions of early childhood. Thus, the erotic image may be switched from the orthodox one of the female being loved by the male to a more complex form called a fetish. The male may fix sexually on an article of clothing, on a specific object or type of behavior, or he may need to change his own gender image in order to achieve erotic arousal. The so-called pedophile fixes on little children, and the gerontophile fixes on old people. Masochists can only have sex associated with pain or humiliation, and sadists must be able to inflict pain on their sexual partner in order to get aroused. Thus, the need for any unusual type of sexual stimulation, from a harmless clothing fetish to a criminal sexual compulsion, is included in paraphilia.

Intersex is a physical condition in which a child is born either with ambiguous genitals that don't clearly identify it as male or female or with genitalia that are the opposite of the baby's true genetic sex. The most fascinating thing about these intersex babies is that they will develop the normal sexual identity of their sex of rearing no matter what their original sexual appearance. A little boy born without a penis who is raised as a girl from earliest infancy develops the normal psychosexual identity of a girl. She has fully feminine traits and habits, and is interested only in males when she grows up, even though she has male chromosomes and started out in life as a boy. The information doctors have obtained from these intersex children has yielded very solid scientific information with which it is possible to make very firm statements now about the development of most of the sexual preferences.

When Does Gender Confusion Start?

What stimulates males to become sexually aroused is not programmed in their genes, nor is it preordained. If it were, any male could be sexually turned on by and fall in love with any female. The heterosexual man's sexual preference is not for all women but for only specific types of women. Each man has developed specific tastes and preferences, and has his own image of the ideal sexual partner. It is perfectly normal for a heterosexual man to be turned on by only a small number of the women he meets.

These erotic visual preferences are no more innate than the language that a person speaks. A child's earliest social experience determines his sexual identity and his image of the preferred sexual partner, just as the language spoken to and around a child will be the one he begins to speak at around eighteen months of age. If in the earliest years of his life a little boy becomes fixed on an image of himself that is confusing, then he may grow up as out of step with his society as the child who is born in a house where no language is spoken or where the language of the country in which he lives is strictly forbidden.

Homosexual and transsexual men can trace their sexual preference back to the earliest recollections of childhood. Instead of having the usual four-year-old's crush on a little girl, they recollect either no such crush or possibly a crush on a little boy instead. At as early as one and a half years of age, instead of walking around in their father's shoes they were walking in their mother's shoes. In kindergarten, they would draw pictures of their mother, or of a woman, instead of a man. Around the so-called latent years, between the ages of six and twelve, they had very few, if any, male friends. They tended to play regularly with the girls, while their male peers fastidiously avoided them. Then, with the hormonal outburst of puberty, they began to find themselves sexually attracted to other boys, they dreamed of boys while having wet dreams, and fantasized about having sexual play with boys when they masturbated. Thus, most homosexuals, transsexuals, and transvestites give a history dating as far into their childhood as the mind can remember.

There are, of course, disagreements among psychologists and psychiatrists regarding the causes of gender confusion. But whatever the cause, there is no controversy on one point: the origins of homosexuality and gender confusion lie very deep in early infancy. They do not simply appear out of nowhere later in life.

Is Gender Confusion Chemical or Genetic in Origin?

As early as 1941 Kinsey reported that injecting male hormone into an animal increases the frequency and intensity of its sexual activity, but does not affect the animal's choice of sexual partner. In human males the intensity of sexual activity is also increased by the administration of testosterone, and there is no effect on the choice of partner; heterosexual men still prefer women and homosexual men still prefer men. If homosexual men are given large doses of testosterone, it only heightens their sexual desire for other men.

Despite some poorly performed studies to the contrary, most scientists now recognize that homosexuals as a group do not have any lower level of male hormone in their system than other men. In fact, there appears to be no hormonal or genetic difference between homosexual and heterosexual men.

Whenever transsexual men are given male hormone in an effort to change their gender identity and to "masculinize" them, all that happens is they become jumpy and nervous, unable to sleep, and depressed. They feel unhappy about the increased beard growth and feel no change whatsoever in their desire to be a woman and have intercourse with men. Furthermore, there are specific clinical conditions in which otherwise normal-appearing men have low testosterone levels, yet these men are rarely homosexuals. Thus despite numerous efforts to put forth a hormonal cause for transsexualism or homosexuality, it appears that these men are clearly not hormonally or genetically different from other men.

Yet there is some controversial evidence that hormonal events occurring while the boy is simply an embryo can partially pre-program his brain for a tendency to gender misidentity. The validity of these studies may determine to a large extent society's view toward homosexuals. Do some children come out of the womb already predestined toward homosexuality, or is it events that occur after they are born that fix their sexual preferences? We really don't know whether sex hormones in the womb have a direct effect on masculinity or femininity of the male embryo's developing brain. But some people think they do. Most of these theories were suggested in the early 1950s and were based on experiments performed on rats, and that is probably where the error lies.

If a newborn female rat is injected with testosterone, later when she grows up her ovaries will fail to ovulate because her brain has been masculinized and will not allow ovulation. Furthermore, if the testicles of a newborn male rat are removed within the first few days of life, when he matures his brain will respond in the same fashion to ovarian hormones as would a normal female rat's brain. Thus if an ovary were transplanted from a female rat into a normal male rat, it would never ovulate. But if an ovary were transplanted into a male rat who had been castrated around the time of birth, the ovary would ovulate.

What about the sexual behavior of these rats when they mature? When a normal male rat is castrated as an adult, he does not behave like a female rat sexually no matter how much female hormone is given him. However, if a male rat is castrated at the time of birth, giving him female hormones as an adult will indeed make him behave sexually as though he were a female rat. Furthermore, if a newborn female rat is injected with testosterone during the first week of life, she will never behave sexually like a normal adult female, despite the fact that her ovaries are producing female hormone. Castrating the male rat after the first week of life, or giving the female rat male hormone after the first week of life, will not in any way change their sexual preference in adulthood. But before the first week of life these hormonal treatments will quite specifically reverse their sexual goals.

The problem with these rat studies is that sexual desire in the female rat is stimulated not by testosterone (as in males) but purely by estrogen, just prior to ovulation. The female rat goes through a period of "heat" just prior to ovulation, when her estrogen level is very high, and it is only during that time that she has any interest in sex. The female rat is strictly turned on by a chemical reaction and nothing else. The rat's mechanism of arousal is incredibly simple as compared to that of the human, which is incredibly complex and controlled mostly by the higher regions of the brain. If the male rat is given testosterone, he wants sex. If the female rat is given estrogen, she wants sex. There is no complex partner-choosing mechanism involved.

Human sexual preference does not seem to be imprisoned by hormonal events, but rather is subject much more to experience and early social conditioning. Homosexuality and gender confusion may be much more possible in the complex social world of humans than in rats. Just because laboratory rats that are given the wrong hormone at birth by some curious scientist developed gender confusion does not mean that some sort of hormonal mix-up in human embryos or newborn infants is responsible for homosexuality.

We know that unlike female rats, human females subjected to high levels of male hormone prior to birth do ovulate when they grow up and have a normal female gender identity. On the other hand, such girls do tend to exhibit a great deal of tomboyish behavior and seem to prefer stereotypically masculine activities. But this tomboyish behavior is a minor event when compared to the fact that such little girls exposed to extremely high levels of male hormone as embryos still grow up to be normal heterosexual women if they are raised unambiguously as girls. Thus, it is possible that prenatal sex hormones may create a *predisposition* toward masculine or feminine behavior, but do not preordain sexual identity or homosexuality. It is the child's entire experience, from the moment he or she leaves the womb, that affects its gender identity.

Some incredibly gross hormonal errors in the human embryo have been proved not to cause homosexual identity or behavior. It is thus highly unlikely that some obscure, subtle hormonal error will have any effect on the child's development as homosexual or heterosexual. Even the slightly tomboyish behavior of girls who obviously were exposed to far too much male hormone in the womb could be explained in other ways. The large clitoris that develops as a result of excessive testosterone in female fetuses might have made the parents somewhat unsure whether their child was a boy or a girl. That slight doubt in the original rearing, prior to the definitive decision that she was a girl, could have been a cause for her subsequent tomboyish behavior.

The postulate that a child is simply "born that way," and that a child's sexual identity is determined by events beyond the parents' control, may be consoling to parents who wonder what they might have done differently. But there isn't any solid scientific evidence to validate this notion. As we will explain in the following two chapters, the scientific evidence is that sexual identity and sexual preferences are determined during the first two years of a child's life, and thus would *appear* to be innate by the time anybody pays attention to them. But they are not innate. They are determined by the social environment to which the child is exposed in the earliest months of life.

Can Sexual Preference Change Later in Life?

One of the greatest fears of many parents is that if their child meets or gets to know a homosexual he might become homosexual himself. Another fear that accompanies this (which can be seen on the face of every housewife whenever a homosexual issue comes up on "The Donahue Show") is that in some way the increasing visibility of homosexuality in recent years will make it easier for young people to slip into it.

The common example of homosexual behavior suddenly appearing in adulthood is, of course, among prisoners. A close look at this situation will give us a better idea of whether homosexuality can begin late in life. It is well known that homosexual behavior occurs in prison. Yet when most prisoners who have practiced homosexuality get out, they return to having sex with women.

We know that when rats are overcrowded experimentally, the lack of living space causes atypical sexual behavior in the males; they begin to make extremely ferocious sexual attacks on females, and homosexual attacks on other, less dominant, males. Still, it is hard for most men to imagine how a heterosexual man can change, even under the stress of being in prison, to being sexually attracted to other men. Yet it happens in rats whose sexuality is an extremely simple chemical event, and in the grizzly experience of the long-term prisoner it seems to occur also. How does it happen?

The key to understanding how a heterosexual man, confined within prison walls with only other men, can begin to engage in homosexual activity is that to him it is a slight improvement over masturbation. Most men in our society, and almost all teenagers, will masturbate when deprived of sexual relations with women. While they are masturbating they are not thinking about their own penis, but are fantasizing that they are having sexual relations with a woman. It is similar with the majority of prisoners engaging in homosexual activity. These men say that while they are having sex with other men they are imagining that they are really having sex with a woman.

This is not to say that there aren't true, obligatory homosexuals in prison. The obligatory homosexual only wants to have sex with other men, and can participate in sex with women only if he is imagining in his fantasy that his partner is truly another man. Thus the obligatory homosexual in prison may be quite delighted to find so many men willing to engage in homosexual activities. But for most other prisoners, homosexuality is simply the best substitute they can find for a woman.

One prison inmate described his conversion to homosexuality and back to heterosexuality in a scientific paper published by Dr. John Money of Johns Hopkins University. The patient had been in jail for eighteen months before ever indulging in sex with another male. He said as time went on "without a woman" he desired a woman so intensely that sometimes he used to watch a man in the shower and imagine it was a naked woman. He said he was shocked to find that as he imagined the man was a naked woman, his penis became erect, and he masturbated. This masturbating in the presence of a naked man led him to realize that "some guys . . . have more a woman's physique, perfect curves from the back, big cheeks. I don't know . . ." He finally approached an inmate he knew was a homosexual, and had sex with him. "I always just pictured him as a woman, a woman I wanted to be with when I was on the outside." In his wet dreams he still imagined having sex with a woman, and his homosexual experience was nothing different for him than a wet dream acted out consciously.

Most of the homosexuality in prison is a brutal affair where one man subjugates another. The majority of men in prison are so firmly heterosexual that they simply would never engage in sex with another man. Yet these men are often attacked by the "gorillas" who want to have sex with something animate, who force themselves to imagine their victims as women, and literally rape them. One prisoner described the absolute horror of men being raped in prison. "It is unbelievable. You can hear the guy hollering and no one doing nothin' about it. . . . I could actually hear the guy crying. Then afterwards he hung himself. The other guy who was raped slashed his wrists."

Apparently it is the "nice-looking guys" with "nice features" who are usually approached for homosexual relations, even if they are completely heterosexual. According to one prisoner, "Governors and legislatures can build walls . . . but they cannot stop men from thinking about sex, from masturbating, nor from other avenues of sexual expression." It is hard for most of us to imagine the barbarian cruelty that can express itself in the unnatural environment of a prison. But the most compelling reflection this casts upon the whole phenomenon of homosexuality is that the non-homosexual man does not become homosexual because he is in prison. He is merely finding another form of masturbation, and his fantasies, which are the indelible clue to his sexual preference, are always about women.

Similarly, when a homosexual tries to have intercourse with a female, he has to imagine that he is in truth having sex with a male in order to do it. Many homosexuals and transsexuals are so culturally keyed into standard values that they suppress their homosexual urge, get married, have a career, and raise children. In order to have sex with his wife, though, a homosexual man must fantasize that he is actually having sex with a man. But eventually, when for one reason or other the stress of the marital relationship becomes too much, he may someday give up his heterosexual relationship to fall in love with another man and have an affair with him. It may appear that this is a case of an adult male switching over from heterosexuality to homosexuality, perhaps influenced by the liberality of our era. But in truth when a man appears suddenly to become a homosexual at a later age, he is finally acting out in reality the fantasies with which he has lived since infancy.

Masters and Johnson recently received a great deal of criticism from knowledgeable members of the scientific community for reporting a high success rate in converting homosexuals to heterosexual life. One reason for this intense criticism was the known fact that erotic preference cannot be changed by voluntary decree or behavioral therapy. Nonetheless, they did seem to have considerable success in helping certain dissatisfied homosexuals change to a heterosexual life-style. The reason for the controversy and the confusion is probably that Masters and Johnson never included in their report any description of the erotic imagery or mental fantasies of the homosexuals who desired to change.

The one unshakable, constant guideline in this controversial area is the content of the man's erotic fantasy. Homosexuals who are dissatisfied with that life-style, and who wish to become heterosexual, can do so only by calling up into their consciousness and utilizing to whatever degree possible the heterosexual imagery they already possess. An obligatory homosexual will never be able to change unless he is able to imagine himself having relations with another man when he is in truth having relations with a woman. But a bisexual individual, that is, a homosexual with some heterosexual erotic imagery, is capable of using that heterosexual eroticism to change his life-style with the aid of counseling if he so desires.

It was once thought that sexual instinct and drive suddenly

arrive at the time of puberty. The hormones turn on, and the child becomes an adolescent full of sexual drives, emotional turmoil, and unpredictability. This is supposedly the time of great volatility in the child's life, and great impressionability, when he might swing in any direction—toward homosexuality, heterosexuality perversion, criminality, or some other kind of antisocial activity of which parents disapprove. But in truth puberty is not the onset of sexuality, or of sexual preference. It is not even the onset of criminality or impressionability. The child's personality, his sex identity, and his entire metaphysical view of life have been firmly established during the important developmental years from birth to age five. From age five to age twelve he is merely consolidating a personality structure that has already been well established.

The burst of hormones that characterizes puberty merely fuels the fire that has already been burning. The mind and body are suddenly activated with sexual desire whose content was programmed years earlier. The little boy going through puberty suddenly has erotic dreams and fantasies that are literally a signature of his own erotic preference. These adolescents do not choose what turns them on. They simply encounter it already established in their mind. Thus, the notion that one can suddenly become a homosexual in adult life, or indeed that he can switch from homosexuality to heterosexuality, is, strictly speaking, not valid. One can modify his behavior because of cultural and personal preferences for a life-style, but he cannot erase that imagery burned indelibly into his brain in the earliest years of his existence.

But we are getting ahead of ourselves. Let's proceed step by step with our knowledge of how gender identity is established. Then we will be able to see how it affects sexual preference in adulthood.

15

Establishment
of Sexual Identity

Stages of Psychosexual Development
from Birth to Twelve Years of Age

Every little event during the earliest months of a child's life has an intense effect on his subsequent personality. From studies of intersex children it is now clear that a child's gender identity as boy or girl begins forming very early in life and is usually well established by the time the child is eighteen months of age. From that time to the onset of puberty, the child is merely consolidating this identity. The specific studies from which this information has been derived will be discussed in detail later in the chapter.

Children appear to be basically unisexual during the first year of life, but sometime after that we see signs of male or female identity in their behavior. A little boy rummaging in his parents' closet usually begins to show a preference for his father's clothes, and will often find a pair of his father's old shoes and try to walk around in them. Although the little boy will usually see more of his mother than his father, after he is about one and a half years old he will show a particular enthusiasm for his father when he comes home. These are typical signs that clearly indicate that the boy has already come to identify with his father.

If a male child prefers to rummage in his mother's closet and wear her shoes or clothes, it may be a very early sign of gender confusion. When such a preference appears after a child is two years old, it is referred to by psychiatrists as cross-dressing. Although a certain amount of cross-dressing can be expected as a normal part of the child's experimentation with gender identity, a consistent preference for the clothes of the mother may be a sign of gender confusion.

The boy's self-concept as male begins to become firmly established by eighteen months of life, and with each succeeding month becomes more and more fixed. It is well known that children begin to establish their sense of self at about the same time that they first begin to speak. That is why native language, accent, and inflection are such an indelible part of character. This self-concept is by definition specific for whether they are boys or whether they are girls. Scientists refer to this most basic self-concept as "core gender identity."

Between the ages of four and six, the little boy who has a firmly established male identity is likely to have a crush on little girls his own age. His relationship to the little girl may be one of admiration from afar, and he is usually entirely too embarrassed to express it very well. But any mother knows about the sweetheart crush that her little four- or five-year-old son has had on at least one girl in his class. This crush occurs in the life of almost every normal little boy, and is not a sign that the boy is a sissy nor of some sort of effeminate development. In fact, it is absolutely normal that he go through this "rehearsal" of falling in love.

Then, between the ages of six and twelve, something very remarkable happens: the little boy loses all interest in girls. This is the so-called latent period, during which boys do not like the activities that girls engage in, and want nothing more than to play with other little boys, usually in rough-and-tumble activities. Although on the surface young boys do not want to have anything to do with girls during this entire period, most adults who can recollect this period of their life remember having some unspoken attraction for girls, coupled with embarrassment and disgust. During this latent period most boys are interested in consolidating their gender identity as males, and any association with females on a peer basis may threaten that self-identity. To some extent this latent period is culturally induced and may not be truly needed to protect a securely established male identity.

As they are entering this latent phase, around age six or seven, boys will demonstrate the importance of their own gender identity by drawing a picture of a person of their own sex when asked to draw a picture in school. In a small number of cases, otherwise normal boys will draw pictures of females, demonstrating that they are attracted to females. But most boys as part of this effort to consolidate their own identity will only draw a picture of other boys or of their father, or someone they imagine to be their father or older brother. During most of their playtime between the ages of six and twelve, boys and girls segregate, as though to further consolidate their gender identities and keep their roles free of mutual contamination.

Then comes adolescence. Many parents have the mistaken view that this is when the child's sexual preference develops. In truth it is the time at which the sexual character, already well established, begins to declare itself. The adolescent boy suddenly finds himself daydreaming about women, having an urge to masturbate, or dreaming of having a beautiful girl in his arms. He is even sometimes awakened in the middle of the night by a wet dream in which he imagines having intercourse with a woman. The adolescent boy makes no decision about this imagery in his dreams or in his fantasies. He has no choice. But if his gender identity was confused by earlier environmental experiences, he will find himself surprised not by erotic fantasies about girls, but rather by erotic fantasies involving other boys. No matter how badly he may want to have the gender identity that he feels would be that of a normal boy, he cannot deny his own history. It is indelibly imprinted on his brain, just as heterosexual preference is imprinted on the brains of other boys.

These patterns of sexual preference and taste are firmly rooted in the basic establishment of our identity, as firmly rooted as our native language, dating back to the earliest months of our existence. Mothers and fathers should know that any child who has gone through the normal psychosexual landmarks from zero to five years of age, and then through a normal latency period from five to twelve years of age, is not suddenly going to become a homosexual.

Gender Identity in Intersex Children

Nowhere is the importance of early environment in the establishment of gender identity more clearly visible than in the cases where children born with ambiguous genitalia are assigned the sex opposite their biological sex. In every case, it is the sex of rearing that these intersex children adopt and carry with them into adulthood. Let's look at a few case histories.

ADRENOGENITAL SYNDROME

Adrenogenital syndrome is a rare condition in which genetically normal little girls produce an excess amount of testosterone. Even while in the mother's womb, the adrenal gland of these girls produces too much male hormone, and because of that they are born with ambiguous genitalia. The clitoris is enlarged so much that it looks like a small penis, and occasionally the vagina is actually fused shut much like the scrotum of a little boy. The excess male hormone production of these little girls can be curbed with small doses of a drug called prednisone. After this drug is administered, the excessive male hormone production ceases and they become normal girls; the clitoris is then rebuilt surgically and the vagina is opened. If a correct diagnosis is made before the age of eighteen months, and the little girl is raised as a little girl, she will grow up to have a normal female sexual identity. Although these girls have had huge amounts of male hormone while they were developing in the womb, they grow up to be normal girls with a normal sexual preference for males, but only if they are raised as girls prior to the age of eighteen months.

If, however, there is some confusion about whether she is a little girl or a little boy, and if this confusion persists past the age of eighteen months, it becomes increasingly difficult for her to establish a female identity. In fact, if it was suddenly determined when she was three years old that she was in truth a girl rather than a boy, the parents would be completely unsuccessful in trying to raise her as a girl.

Interestingly, most of these adrenogenital girls exhibit tomboyish behavior as they grow up, prefer to play with boys their age rather than girls, shun dolls and "feminine" skills, and seem in many ways to display what our culture views as a masculine type of gender behavior. Although a small percentage of these women become homosexuals, the vast majority of these little girls born with genitals that look almost male, and who had tremendous amounts of male hormone circulating in their systems from the earliest possible age, nonetheless develop normal female identities if they are raised as girls from the earliest months of life. They eventually fall in love with men, marry, and are firm heterosexuals.

Some little girls with adrenogenital syndrome have such severely high testosterone levels that when they are born they have a completely normal penis rather than an enlarged clitoris. They look just like little boys with undescended testicles, and in this case the doctor will frequently miss the diagnosis that it is a girl. Such a child will usually be raised as a boy until puberty. Some doctors have been tempted in the past to reassign these boys as girls, remove their penis, open their vagina, and make them anatomically normal females, capable of having children. But it doesn't work. Their gender identity as males has already been firmly fixed, and any attempt to reassign them as females after the age of two years will fail. Little boys who are raised as little boys stay little boys.

TESTICULAR FEMINIZATION

There is a small group of genetically normal little boys whose testicles produce normal amounts of male hormone, but whose bodies are completely unresponsive to the effects of the testosterone. Therefore these little boys never develop a penis or any external male genitalia. They have two normal testicles located in the abdomen, but otherwise they look exactly like little girls. They do not have a scrotum, but rather have female labia. The clitoris never enlarged, and the scrotum never fused in the middle, thus leaving an open vagina. The small quantity of estrogen produced normally by the testicles is enough to feminize the body contours and induce these genetic males to grow normal feminine breasts at puberty. In fact, these little boys are completely indistinguishable from little girls, and are always raised as little girls. They always develop a normal female gender identity and when they grow up desire a male sexual partner.

Occasionally in these cases the clitoral organ is just large enough that the physician makes the error of deciding the baby should be declared a boy. The doctor may try surgically to make the clitoris look as much like a penis as possible, and the parents may raise the child as a boy. Yet because the body tissues are inadequately responsive to testosterone, such a boy never really develops a male body. He develops female contours, breasts, and never develops a large enough penis to be considered usable for intercourse. Interestingly, this sexually inadequate male develops a completely normal male gender identity in spite of all these physical obstacles, and in spite of a body and brain incapable of being masculinized by testosterone. After two years of age it is too late to make him a girl. His identity is indelibly established. But this man imprisoned in a feminine body structure demonstrates the profound effect of rearing and environment over early or late hormonal events.

SEXUAL REASSIGNMENT
AFTER DAMAGE TO THE PENIS

In one particularly unusual case, the entire penis of one of a pair of normal, identical twin boys was burned off at seven months of age by an improperly performed circumcision. The little boy with the destroyed penis was then reassigned as a girl since there was nothing that could be done to restore the lost penis. He underwent reconstructive surgery to create a vagina and his testicles were removed. By seventeen months of age the parents were firmly determined to raise the little boy as a girl, changing the name, clothing, and hair style, as well as having all of the appropriate reconstructive surgery to make it a female. They reared the one twin who still had his penis and testicles as a normal boy, and the other twin as a normal girl. Eventually the little girl developed a normal female gender identity, and her brother developed a normal male gender identity. The mother reports that the boy clearly imitated the father's behavior and the girl copied her own behavior. The girl wanted dolls and feminine games, while the boy wanted a garage with cars and tools. The girl had many tomboyish traits, but because of the cues and reinforcements of parental rearing, this little boy who once had a penis became a normal little girl. If the penis is destroyed at twenty-four months of life, however, it is too late to try to rear the boy as a girl. Even without a penis, he is mentally fixed as a boy by the time he is two years old, and nothing can change it.

THE BOY WITH A MICROPENIS

A similar situation to the one just discussed occurs when a normal baby boy is born with a micropenis. Such a penis will never grow to a normal adult size, and many of these boys are reassigned as girls. As long as the reassignment takes place before eighteen months of age, it is successful; despite male chromosomes and male hormones in embryonic life and infancy, the boy can grow up to be a normal girl. But if there is any ambiguity in the parents' view of whether it is a boy or a girl, or if the reassignment of sex takes place after eighteen months, success becomes increasingly difficult.

Sometimes a boy who is born with a micropenis is raised as a boy. When he goes through puberty, his little penis will hardly develop at all, and it will be completely inadequate for intercourse when he is an adult. We are not talking about a short penis of two inches in length, but rather a half-inch penis. When the boy goes through adolescence and younger adulthood, he feels completely inadequate as a man, and he may reflect on how much better it might have been to have been changed into a girl. But try as he may to think about having any kind of sex-change surgery, the boy simply cannot alter his sexual identity. When he masturbates, his fantasies are those of a boy with a normal penis having sex with a girl. Despite the difficulties facing him because of his tiny sex organ, such a boy is a normal heterosexual male because that is the way he was programmed in his first several years of life.

MATCHED HERMAPHRODITES

The most impressive proof of the effect of environment and rearing on sexual identity and gender differentiation comes from observations of matched pairs of hermaphrodites. A hermaphrodite is a child who is born with both an ovary and a testicle, and thus with both male and female genitals. The decision as to whether this child should be raised as a boy or a girl is usually quite arbitrary. Researchers have kept track of hermaphrodites who have the same unusual combination of male and female structures, some of whom were raised as boys from earliest childhood, and others as girls. So long as the parents have absolutely no doubt or ambiguity as to whether they feel they are raising a son or a daughter, the way they raise them is the way they grow up.

If the parents are in doubt about the baby's "authentic" sex, they may watch the baby's behavior with overabundant vigilance, looking intensely for any sign to resolve their doubt. In doing so, they transmit mixed signals, and the child may not then be able to establish firmly its sexual identity. Any hermaphrodite child who decides later in life that it was assigned wrongly as a boy or a girl can always trace this problem back to an uncertainty on the part of the parents as to what he or she really was or should have been.

KLINEFELTER'S SYNDROME
AND BOYS WITHOUT TESTICLES

Some men are born with normal male genitals, but instead of having XY chromosomes (as do normal males), they have what is called XXY chromosomes; that is, they have one extra female chromosome. The testicles of these men usually make only a small amount of testosterone, and no sperm at all. Men with this condition (called Klinefelter's syndrome) are usually partly eunuch, and certainly have never had a normal amount of testosterone circulating in their bodies. Yet in almost all cases patients with Klinefelter's syndrome are not homosexuals or transsexuals. Because they were raised as boys they have the identity of boys and the sexual desire of boys, albeit somewhat minimized by their relatively low testosterone levels. Replacement of testosterone in these men returns their libido to normal.

An even more convincing case of sex of rearing overriding physical shortcomings is the little boy born without testicles. In essentially every case boys with this condition develop normal male sexual identity. Their complete lack of testosterone production in no way prevents them from growing up as normal boys with normal sexual desires. If their parents are confused about whether or not they are boys, that is a different story. But if these children are raised unambiguously as boys, then that is the way they will view themselves.

"PENIS AT TWELVE" SYNDROME

There is a very rare condition, scientifically referred to as 5 alpha reductase deficiency, but otherwise known as the "penis at twelve" syndrome. In this case genetically normal XY boys with normal testicles have a reduced (rather than absent) responsiveness of the body tissues to testosterone because their cells cannot convert testosterone to its active form. They are born with severe ambiguity of the external genitals and many of the infants are thought to be girls at birth and are raised as girls. Then at the time of puberty, with the tremendous increase in testosterone production, the body responds by actually masculinizing. The clitoris-like phallus grows into a normal penis, the voice deepens, a male muscular pattern develops, testes suddenly descend from the abdomen into the scrotum, and these boys have erections and even ejaculate. They are essentially normal boys, who are born looking somewhat like females, are raised as girls, and who then suddenly at puberty grow a penis, and find out that they are boys.

This is a genetically transmitted but rare disease. There is a particular family of these cases found in a remote village of the Dominican Republic that has been studied extensively. This study has supposedly challenged the otherwise unshakable conclusion that the sex of rearing and environmental factors after birth are the critical components in determining sex identity. Most of the little boys in the Dominican Republic, who were raised as girls, and then suddenly at puberty found they had a penis, switched their gender identity from girls to boys. The authors of this study concluded that, contrary to almost all of the other studies available, the effects of testosterone were more important in the determination of gender identity than the effect of the children's being reared as girls.

But there are several objections to such an interpretation of this study. The female identity of these children may not have really been fixed because of early ambiguity on the part of their parents. Certainly these little boys did not look like normal little girls, but rather had very ambiguous genitalia with a huge clitoris which could easily be thought of as a penis. There are other cases of intersex children who changed their sex of assignment, but in all of these cases there was uncertainty in their original environment as to what sex they were. Ambiguity in the parents' minds can be transmitted to the child, and this ambiguity can go only one way—toward the opposite sex. When there is sufficient doubt about whether the child is really a boy or a girl during the first one and a half to two years of life, there is a chance that the child will ultimately decide to change its identity later.

There are also cases of the "penis at twelve" syndrome where the child was truly raised unambiguously as a girl. In these cases, when the girl became virile at age fourteen and looked masculine, it did not change her female gender identity. She was horrified. She wanted nothing more than to get rid of her new-found maleness and to continue living as a female. The authors of the study from the Dominican Republic admitted that these little "girls" knew that something was wrong at an early age, because they knew they had testicles. It is impossible to be sure that they were truly raised as normal girls. There had to be some ambiguity in their minds during childhood about what sex they were. Thus, in the Dominican Republic study, it is likely that when these little girls suddenly grew long penises and developed normal maleness, it was a great relief to them because all along they must have suspected they were boys.

Interestingly, in the few cases of "penis at twelve" syndrome where the little boy was unambiguously reared as a little girl, the sudden release of male hormone at puberty brought out feminine rather than masculine sexual arousal. When such girls went through their "masculine" puberty, the little girls experienced erotic attraction toward boys, and no erotic attraction toward girls. The images that stimulated erotic arousal developed independently of the girls' hormones, and were completely determined by biography. Thus, despite the disturbance created by this fascinating study from the Dominican Republic, the overwhelming weight of evidence is that even in these cases it is the environment of rearing that determines for the most part one's ultimate psycho-sexual orientation, gender identity, and sexuality preference.

Imprinting

If sex reassignment is made after a child is two years of age, it will not work. A clean break with the originally assigned sex can only be made prior to this critical age. This early indelible fixation of identity is called imprinting, a concept originally discovered in the 1930s by the famous biologist Konrad Lorenz. Lorenz discovered that when he squatted in front of newly hatched mallard ducklings, and removed their mother, so that he was the first thing the ducklings saw when their eyes opened, the birds followed him with the same devotion as though he were their true mother. Once this imprinting occurred it was completely indelible and unmodifiable. Even when the ducklings' true mother was returned to them, they would only follow Lorenz. After he imprinted his image on newly hatched jackdaws in the same fashion, when they grew to sexual maturity these little birds would court only human beings. These little birds literally thought of themselves not as jackdaws but as humans.

A mallard duck that is placed with geese right after hatching thinks that it is a goose rather than a mallard duck and will only choose a goose as its sexual mate. Furthermore, if a male mallard duck is exposed only to other male mallard ducks upon hatching and never sees female ducks, it will become fixated exclusively on a male as a potential mating partner. Both such "homosexual" ducks will react to each other as though the other were a female.

The homosexually imprinted duckling will not usually mate with a partner that was among the group it hatched with. If the male duckling is reared almost exclusively in the company of other males, but there are one or two females around, then the duck becomes only partially homosexual. When it grows up and reaches sexual maturity, it may show a homosexual mating preference or a heterosexual preference. Some of these homosexually imprinted male ducks will only show a brief homosexual preference and will eventually pick only female ducks for sexual partners. But once these male ducklings have been imprinted to think that their sexual preference is for other males, it becomes impossible to induce them experimentally to reverse their behavior pattern.

It is fascinating that female mallard ducklings do *not* show this same early vulnerability to homosexual or cross-species imprinting as males. Whether or not females are hatched in the presence of only females, when they grow to their sexual maturity they will still pick males as their sexual partners. This bears a familiar resemblance to the human situation, in which homosexuality and errors of gender identification are at least four times more common in men than in women. The male's whole psychosexual development is much more of a frail, confused, and potentially vulnerable process than that of the female.

Imprinting in human beings is, of course, much more complicated than in these simpler animals. The diverse variety of cues that the child receives during the critical period of the first eighteen months of life are almost impossible to analyze. But whatever these specific cues are, it is clear that the parents' view of the child and their interaction with the child indelibly record and print into the baby's brain, in ways so complex and so subtle as to defy analysis, just exactly what sex he or she is.

Parental Behavior and the Child's Gender Identity

Certainly it is easy enough to recognize that the little boy identifies with his father as a role model in establishing his sex identity. But that is certainly too simple a view. Many women who rear their sons alone without a husband have no problem in their child's developing a normal male identity, and their sons do not usually become homosexuals. Furthermore, having a strong father to identify with does not necessarily prevent the little boy from misidentifying himself as a girl. If his father is so brutally strong and unfeeling that the boy shies away from any emotional attachment to him, he may be an impossible figure to identify with, and once again gender identity will go astray. Many parents worry that if the male parent shows a tremendous amount of affection and love toward the male son that this might encourage a homosexual predisposition on the part of the child. Nothing could be further from the truth.

The ordinary infant is exposed to both men and women in his environment very much like the child of an immigrant family is exposed to two different languages. The child of the immigrant has a remarkable ability to separate these two entirely different sets of language stimuli that he receives at the earliest age and to choose as his native language the language of the country in which he resides, even though it is not the native language of his parents. Similarly the child establishes his sex identity through two major processes. He identifies with a person of the same sex, and complements the parent of the opposite sex.

The child assimilates in his mind the two sets of behavior that he observes, the behavior of females and the behavior of males. It does not particularly matter whether the father enjoys certain activities that our culture says are not typically "masculine," or whether the mother enjoys certain activities that our culture has not categorized as "feminine." The content of these masculine or feminine roles is not nearly so important as the clear-cut lack of ambiguity transmitted to the child. If the child receives messages from a liberated household that it is acceptable for the father to do the dishes and for the mother to go to work, that will not predispose him toward becoming a homosexual or having gender confusion. It doesn't matter if the father is a chef and the mother is a construction worker. The cues that the child receives in his earliest months and years of life will be far more subtle, far more numerous, and far more complex than that.

The child assimilates in his brain all of the different behaviors of the father-figure and mother-figure in his life, just as the immigrant child assimilates the two different languages that his ears are constantly bombarded with. In accordance with whether he is reared as male or as female, he will code the behavior of the like sex parent as positive and the opposite sex parent as negative. Father and mother may have remarkably similar attitudes and liberated views of their responsibility toward society. The important thing is for the infant to perceive that the male cues that surround him are positive and that the female cues complement those male cues.

From the very earliest seconds of life, one of the first questions that is always asked about the baby is whether it is a boy or a girl. This pervasive factor in human culture everywhere is the best testimony we have to the fact that in many ways far beyond our conscious power we treat little boys and little girls differently. This viewpoint on the part of the parents is unshakable and cannot be hidden. Indeed, even the parents' love for each other has a positive effect on the baby and helps him or her form a proper identity as boy or girl. When the little baby sees that the interaction between the father and mother is a healthy one, then no matter how similar and equal their views of life and responsibility, the child will view them as different and will automatically program himself or herself toward identifying with the parent of the same sex.

By two years of age, children already show a strong preference for playmates of their own sex, and by age three boys are well advanced in their preference for "masculine" toys and male playmates. Little boys three years of age never want to play with dolls, and little girls three years of age are not interested in what the boys are interested in. Once they have established their gender identity, their particular behavior within that identity depends a good deal upon their playmates and the entire society around them. If a boy happens to show an interest in cooking at age five, perhaps because his father likes to cook and to help around the house, this does not make him a sissy nor does it inflict any harm upon his sense of identity as a male. However, if the child's father despises cooking and housework, and if all his peers have similar feelings, but the little boy for some reason prefers to play with dolls and to help his mother in the kitchen, this would be a strong sign that the boy's gender identity is miscued.

It is important that both the father and the mother give the child consistent cues. If the father feels that boys should engage only in rough-and-tumble athletic events and that girls should remain neatly and passively content to do kitchen chores, and if the mother has the opposite view that girls should be able to go out and play baseball and that boys should help more in the kitchen, these discordant messages that father and mother are giving the child do not complement each other, and can confuse his developing sense of self. If the parents are giving discordant or confusing cues to the child, it would probably be better for the child to have only one parent.

Nonetheless, it is preferable for children to have models of both sexes in their immediate environment so that they can learn to identify with one model and complement the behavior of the other. If there is no man in the house, it is helpful for the boy to try to identify with an uncle, a brother, or even a television hero who represents an image of manhood that the mother respects. If the mother does not respect the image of manhood that the men around the child represent, than he will get a confusing series of crossing cues that may lead to problems. Children with the severest gender identity problems, the transsexuals, almost always come from households where no divorce occurred, where the parents are clearly giving discordant signals, where identification with the father is next to impossible, and where the marriage, as intolerable as it is, somehow or other holds together and completely destroys the little boy's efforts to assimilate and segregate his male and female cues successfully.

If a little boy's father rejects him, if his older brother rejects him, and if he gets his only love from his mother and his younger sister, it is very possible that he will interpret his sexual identity as female. It matters not that his father is a strong figure or even an admirable one in the society they live in. The point is that the boy failed to receive love and attention from male figures in his environment and received his only love and attention from females.

A little baby usually displays combinations of masculine and feminine behavior. A male baby receives approval for male-oriented behavior, or disapproval for female-type behavior. It is in this way that a child's mannerisms develop. For example, little boys often expend an incredible amount of energy. It is not really known why it is that boys tend to be more energetic and rough in their play than girls. It may be cultural or it may be innate. But it is very understandable that some parents might react to that type of behavior as though it were hyperactive and certainly annoying to the busy father who has other things on his mind. Such negative reactions to boyish behavior from a father too preoccupied to tolerate it could lead the boy to explore different types of behavior in order to get a more favorable response. This is not to say that a hyperactive boy, ignored by his father, will become a homosexual, since by the time the child is old enough to be this energetic his gender identity is already fairly well established. But a boy whose frenetic activity is received by his father with disfavor may explore other, less conventional mannerisms in his attempts to find parental approval.

Puberty and Falling in Love

Prior to puberty, the boy has gone through all sorts of rehearsals of falling in love, but now the real thing is about to develop. The motors of his sex drive are finally about to turn on and release the sexual identity that was established long before. The boy experiences erotic daydreams, and eventually has wet dreams at night while imagining intercourse with a female.

But the boy destined to be a homosexual finds at puberty that his erotic fantasies and his wet dreams, instead of involving girls, are directed toward other men or boys. He experiences a frightening discordance between the gender identity that he might like to think of himself as having and what in truth he holds within. He cannot by any willful act change the imagery of his dreams or fantasies.

A lot is happening sexually during the years preceding puberty to consolidate the sexual identity that the child has earlier established. Dr. John Money of Johns Hopkins University has pointed out that "privacy" is probably a better term than latency for these prepubertal years. It is a period when sexuality is not overtly expressed. The child is quietly consolidating his own sexual identity and complementing that of the other sex. It is an important period of preparation for the explosive unleashing of erotic desire in puberty. Without the establishment of a proper psychosexual foundation prior to puberty, adolescence can be a confusing and sexually destructive time to the teenager who has not prepared himself with the proper developmental milestones earlier.

The very expression "falling in love" sounds sentimental and almost embarrassing in the cynical age in which we live. In truth, falling in love is a scientifically observable phenomenon that is rather peculiar to humans and which is of immense biologic importance to our survival as a species. In a sense, falling in love is another example of "imprinting." There is a tremendous amount of variation in the features of different individuals that are more or less likely to turn us on. Our preference for specific types of individuals has been programmed unwittingly years earlier, long before adolescence. Adolescence and growing up is simply a time of fine-tuning our psychosexual judgments about potential partners, but it is not a time in which our basic preference patterns for a partner undergo a radical change. Love at first sight is a real phenomenon in which certain visual cues immediately evoke a gigantic reservoir of emotions and feelings passed on from the earliest years of our lives. This huge emotional release is not always consistent with other cues received from the individual as the relationship progresses. But it is surprising how frequently a first impression is a valid one.

It is evidently impossible to fall in love with any individual with whom one has been raised up to age five. Studies from the Israeli kibbutzim have demonstrated that not a single marriage ever took place between two people who grew up close together in the same community for the first five years of life. Close proximity and friendship in these early years seem to rule out a subsequent love relationship. This may be Nature's way of guarding against incestuous love affairs. The intimacy of the close relationship in the earliest years seems to leave an imprint which, though helpful as a rehearsal for falling in love later on with a person of the opposite sex, literally prevents one from falling in love with the rehearsal mate of early life.

The teenage years are filled with many episodes of "falling in love," and the young man is well known for his propensity to fall in and out of love with great rapidity. Eventually in the human animal a permanent pair-bonding does occur. In this case, after the initial explosion of "love" wears off, the couple then find themselves in a calmer, more stable situation where they remain powerfully stimulated by each other sexually and mentally over a prolonged period of time. It is this human characteristic that ultimately results in the strong family bond which may be responsible more than anything else for the special supremacy of human beings on the evolutionary scale.

Falling in love is Nature's way of keeping a man and woman united long enough for their sexual bond to be joined by parental love and thus ensure the proper care and protection of the young. In laboratory rodents, the animals from whom so much of the hormonal predetermination theories have derived, mating behavior results from hormonal factors alone. It is only in the higher primates, and particularly in humans, that personal partner preference comes into play and where sexual preference is not just an automatic reaction to a hormonal injection, but rather a mental event which is only supported, but not directed, by hormones.

16

Transsexualism
and Homosexuality

*What Is a Transsexual and How Is
He Different from a Homosexual?*

Transsexualism is the most extreme type of sexual misidentification. Imagine an individual who thinks of himself as completely and totally a woman in every respect, who desires to be loved sexually as a woman, but who is trapped inside the body of a man. This is exactly the way the transsexual looks at himself. He was born a genetically normal, hormonally normal, physically normal male, but because of the way in which he was brought up, from the very earliest months of his life, he has behaved as though he were a girl and has thought of himself as a girl. A transsexual is not a homosexual and would be offended if referred to as one. A transsexual does not want to have sex with homosexual men or with other transsexual men.

The transsexual despises his genitals and does not want to use them. He doesn't want to masturbate and he doesn't want any partner to touch his sex organs. In fact, he despises his erections, and would prefer having no libido rather than a libido that results in anything resembling a male erection. While the transsexual prefers a male sexual partner in his sexual imagery, overt sexuality plays a very minor role in his life. By contrast, the homosexual has erotic needs and is quite delighted to use his genitals in making love with other men. He views himself as a man, but his sexual preference is for other men. The transsexual views himself as a woman, and his sex organs are an incredible impediment to him.

Many transsexuals go through an early part of their lives trying to be heterosexual, because of a strong desire to have a family and children. The only way a transsexual man is able to have sex with his wife is by fantasizing that he is not a male having sex with a female, but rather that he is a female having sex with a male. This is not much different from a homosexual who accomplishes heterosexual intercourse by imagining that his partner is a male. If any of this seems inconceivable, one need only recognize how common it is for a heterosexual man who is bored with his sexual partner to imagine that he is having sex with a *Playboy* centerfold.

The mental erotic imagery always tells the true story. It explains the seemingly confusing occurrence of a normal husband with a family who suddenly one day decides that he wants to become a woman. In such cases, the man's mental imagery from early childhood has been that he is a woman, and his mental fantasies have always involved sexual attraction, as a woman, to other men.

The most famous transsexual was Christine Jorgensen. Her story was so popularized that long before sex-change clinics opened in America, her name was almost a household word representing the man who successfully changed to a woman. Interestingly, Christine Jorgensen's case came up long before doctors understood anything about transsexualism. Christine Jorgensen was thought to be a homosexual man who suffered from his homosexual impulses, and who wanted to be rid of them. The original intention of the doctors treating Christine Jorgensen in Denmark was not to change him into a woman, but rather to relieve him of his erotic desires, which led him into activity that was socially and culturally unacceptable. Christine Jorgensen, of course, did want to change his sex to female, but the medical team treating him simply regarded him as a homosexual. It had no intention originally of performing a sex-change operation.

In Denmark at that time homosexuals were regarded as a suffering people whose sex drive was not normal. Homosexuals also accepted this attitude and generally accepted the treatment of castration. The philosophy of this treatment was that if the libido could be reduced it would calm the person down so much that he would not desire homosexual activity anymore. So when Christine Jorgensen asked to be castrated, the doctors accommodated him. It was only later that it became apparent that this was not simply a case of castrating a homosexual to relieve him of his sexual desire, but rather that it led to an actual sex reversal, so that this man who wanted to lead the life of a woman could finally do so.

Danish physicians who have now performed the sex-change operation on a very large number of transsexuals subsequent to Christine Jorgensen feel that this is not a simple answer to the problem. It is simply palliative. Only about 10 percent of patients requesting the sex-change operation seem to be helped by it. Still, most of those who undergo surgery in a carefully planned program feel better after the operation than before, and feel that they are at least a step closer to solving the incredible contradiction with which their early rearing has forced them to live. The Danish physicians performing this surgery feel that they are helping these people, but that no one should be misled into thinking that these patients really feel they have truly changed their sex and are finally concordant with their fantasies.

But no other treatment at all is available. No amount of psychotherapy can make these transsexuals happy about being men. The Danish doctors feel that transsexual men live more in a world of fantasy than in reality, and their ability to establish genuine, mutual relationships is rigid and limited. Even after the sex-change operation, this rigidity will not be easily overcome. Most of the Danish doctors who treat these patients feel that for the majority of transsexuals there is simply no hope. No matter what is done, it is likely to be wrong. It would be far better to help parents understand just how this gender confusion occurs, because prevention is so much more effective than treatment.

Sex Reversals in the Animal World

All birds are potential hermaphrodites. Female birds normally develop only one ovary, the left one. All they have on the right side is an old remnant of a gonad that is completely inactive. However, if the left ovary of a hen is removed, she suddenly becomes transformed anatomically and behaviorally into a rooster. When the left ovary is removed, the small rudiment of a gonad on the right grows suddenly into a testicle. The same thing occurs with ducks. Thus a genetically female bird may undergo a complete sex reversal to a male if for some reason her single ovary is destroyed. A hen that has been laying eggs may change into a rooster.

Frogs, toads, newts, and salamanders can be completely sex-reversed by incubating the fertilized egg in small amounts of hormone. These sex reversals are so complete that genetic females can develop fully functional testicles, produce sperm, and these males can then mate with normal females to produce only female offspring. The same bisexuality and sex reversals are found in fish. Newly hatched goldfish can be transformed either to all-female broods when estrogens are added to the water or to all-male broods when testosterone is added.

There is an interesting species of coral reef fish in which all the juveniles mature as females, but a few of those females later transform spontaneously into males. Loss of a single male from this group of female-dominated fish results in the sex reversal of one of the female fish in the group within less than a week. When these fish run out of their limited supply of males, they just make another one. A boundless variation in sex differences in the animal kingdom shows the remarkable adaptability of various species to the particular problems of survival they face.

Is variability in human sexual preference then somehow similar to the adaptations of the coral reef fish, or of the sea anemone, which can change its sexual identity back and forth according to the demands of the environment? Probably not. The single most important characteristic of human life is that humans are a highly social species, and it is our ability to interact in extremely complex ways that has pulled us out of the saltwater. It seems quite unlikely that human transsexualism is some vestige of adaptation to the environment that might have been made far back in history. What then is it that happens to some humans that makes them develop a sexual identity that is the reverse of their physical identity?

What Makes a Little Boy Grow Up to Be a Transsexual?

The history of every single transsexual dates back to earliest childhood. The commitment to change sex is so powerful that for years some scientists speculated that it was simply an innate and unexplainable quirk in these men. But careful psychoanalytic studies probing deep into the childhood of transsexuals have now led to the conclusion that there is a typical, repeatable type of history, beginning at infancy, that accounts for this extreme sexual confusion.

According to Dr. Robert Stoller of the UCLA Department of Psychiatry, who has studied large numbers of these men, the fathers and mothers of these children always displayed a typical pattern that was quite different from fathers and mothers of any other group of children. Dr. Stoller noted that the parents of these boys impinged upon their infant sons with a specific style that forced them to develop in a feminine way, whether consciously or unconsciously. He found that transsexualism always started in the earliest months of childhood, and that it is most likely to occur when a dominant woman is joined with a passive noncommunicating man in an intolerable, empty marriage.

The couple typically decides not to divorce and permits the weakness of their marriage to be seen openly by the child. The father in this marriage can cope with the situation only by being absent, particularly during the infancy and childhood of his son. The wife manages by letting the husband be absent, and comforting herself in continual depression, deriving solace by having an unusually close and totally possessive relationship with her infant son. Stoller defines the typical mother of these transsexuals as a woman who prefers male clothes, looks drab to the extreme in appearance, has a complete lack of need for any heterosexual activity, and who finally entered into a completely passionless marriage.

These mothers never let go of their infant son, day or night, from his infancy into childhood. The mother never lets the baby boy cry, and sleeps with him to prevent him from ever screaming. She feels that as long as she is with her son to the exclusion of everyone else, her boy is happy. She concentrates totally upon him, and nothing else, and her little boy identifies with her completely. He feels himself as a female despite the fact that his senses tell him that he is anatomically a male. In one case, the family arrangement was so bizarre that the child who eventually became a transsexual slept with his mother in one bed, the father and brother slept in another bed, and the two sisters slept in a third bed.

Of course, all mothers of infants are extremely close physically in the first few months of life. This is not only normal but it is essential and important. But when this interaction excludes males and continues unchanged for years, that is when the problem develops. Transsexuals are usually either an only son or the youngest son. The arrival of another baby after a year or two necessarily redirects the mother's attention and this leaves the little boy on his own somewhat more. But if he is the youngest child, or an only child, the mother is able to spend literally all of her time with him, and focus completely upon him.

In most cases of transsexualism, the father was absent most of the time and there was no admirable male figure for the boy to focus upon. The father was either out of town, or away at business in the evenings or during the days. Sometimes he would only get home after the child had gone to bed. Often when he was home on the weekends he would be totally isolated from the family so he could enjoy his various hobbies by himself. Frequently the husband had alcoholic problems or would come home late from a bar. The child had no sense of companionship from the father, and no reason whatsoever either to admire or to identify with him.

In none of the transsexual cases that were studied did the marriage of the transsexual's parents result in divorce. Probably a divorce would have been better, because then there might conceivably have been an opportunity for other male figures to enter the baby's life. But the presence of a totally inadequate father prevented such relationships and there was nothing in the mother's behavior that would complement or encourage male identification on the part of the child. The baby could have developed a normal male gender identity without necessarily having a man to model after, but to do so he would need complementary approval from his mother for male-oriented behavior. He never got that approval, and that, coupled with the lack of any positive male to identify with, led to complete confusion of his sexual identity.

Dr. Stoller makes a rather powerful thesis on the basis of extensive studies that the boy's gender identity is not significantly affected by genetic, hormonal, or physiological phenomena. His bluntly stated theory is that "the degree of femininity as it develops in a boy, and the forms it takes, vary according to (not approximately) what is done to him in earliest childhood." While this statement may be extreme—it is impossible to quantitate "degree of femininity"—it is essentially correct in attributing gender identity to influences on the child in early infancy.

It is very difficult to identify specifically the ways in which the mother of the transsexual may have led to the child's gender confusion. The woman who wears pants and who likes to go to football games should not worry that she is at risk of creating a transsexual son. The exact sensations that she transmits to the infant regarding her own fundamental attitudes about sexual identity are difficult to define, and she can't really control them consciously. But they determine completely the little boy's masculinity or femininity.

I dwell on the published psychoanalytical studies of these transsexual men in great detail because it is the most extreme example of gender confusion. As such it is simpler and easier to understand. Although transsexuals are rare in our society, homosexuality is common. It is often easier to understand the extreme case, however rare it may be, and from that to gain some idea about the more common situation, which is usually a more delicate blend than the extreme. Most of our knowledge of homosexuality has derived from our understanding of transsexualism. Scientific viewpoints on what causes homosexuality and what, if anything, can be done for homosexuals either to improve their homosexual love life or help them change to heterosexual behavior, or indeed to prevent the development of homosexuality in today's youngsters, are a bit controversial. But viewpoints on the transsexual are not so disputable, and the development of transsexualism is much more clearly understood than that of homosexuality. Now we will try to extend our knowledge to the subject of homosexuality. Hopefully this insight will not only make life more tolerable for homosexuals, but will educate and ease the minds of those who are fearful of it.

Homosexuality

Talking to homosexual men about their childhood always reveals that their sexual attraction to other men dates as far back as they can remember. Homosexual men typically have a hard time remembering any father figure with whom they identified, and they usually recall regarding themselves as different from other boys, "an inadequate boy," or "a boy but not a real boy." They were some unreal version of a boy with no male figure in their life whom they could love and admire. Homosexuals do not recall ever having had the typical kindergarten or preschool crush on some little girl; by the time of first grade they might have even had a crush on a little boy. They would never mention this attraction to anyone, and usually would try to suppress or silence the feeling. When asked to draw a picture in kindergarten or first grade, they would almost never draw the figure of a father or any man, unless it was a man to whom they were sexually attracted. During the so-called latent period, between the ages of six and twelve, when most boys are consciously avoiding little girls and playing together in activities that consolidate their identity as boys, the homosexual is actually trying to figure out why he feels different from other boys. The homosexual boy is not necessarily playing exclusively with little girls, but sometimes boys who grow up to be homosexuals do avoid other boys in the same way boys who grow up to be heterosexual avoid little girls.

Effeminate behavior is not necessarily a clue to homosexuality. In fact, most homosexuals are not outwardly effeminate, and most homosexuals are not attracted to effeminate men. Effeminacy is not truly feminine behavior, but rather a caricature of feminine behavior. It is an unreal pretense toward being female, and as such it is just another signal of confusion in sexual identity.

But parents of a boy who has had all of the early landmarks of a normal psychosexual development, such as walking in his father's shoes, rushing to greet daddy when he comes home, having a crush on a little girl at age four or five, drawing a picture of daddy in kindergarten or first grade exercises, and finally going into the latency period, where he will have nothing to do with girls from the age of six to twelve, need not fear that suddenly at puberty he will become a homosexual.

The only prospective scientific study following little boys with severe gender confusion into adulthood was performed by Dr. John Money at Johns Hopkins University. His study links confusion of gender identity in the early childhood of little boys who at first seem to be transsexual to the later development of homosexuality. Eleven little boys were referred to him twenty years earlier because of effeminate behavior, a desire to dress in girls' clothes, or an overt statement of wanting to be a girl. These eleven boys all seemed to be future transsexuals, men who think of themselves as women. But twenty years later, all of these little boys ultimately had become homosexuals. They did not become transsexuals. Over the years they lost their desire to become females and ultimately established a male gender identity, but they retained their image of sexual attraction to other males.

Eight out of the eleven boys had a great preference for their mothers, and none of the eleven showed any preference for his father. Although there was no overt homosexuality or effeminacy in any of the fathers, there was clearly a difficulty in the children's relationship with them. Male identity clearly develops out of an attempt to model after a parent of our own sex. The end result of the parental relationships in each of these cases was the boy's difficulty in identifying with a male figure.

It might seem that these boys would have grown up to become transsexuals and request sex-change operations, but none of them did. In fact, all eleven ultimately became homosexuals. Over the years they lost their childhood desire to become females, and established male gender identities. The sexual fantasies of these men in adulthood are clearly homosexual and completely concordant with their homosexual behavior. Most little boys who state a wish to become girls will probably not grow up as transsexuals. Their male identity, though weak in childhood, will eventually become firmly established, even though their sexual preference remains for other males. In little boys who grow up to be transsexuals, i.e., men who view themselves as women, the relationships at home that led to the total absence of male identification were similar to but just more extreme than in the case of homosexuals.

In between the homosexual and the heterosexual boy is the less clear-cut case of the boy who may be attracted either to boys or girls, the so-called bisexual. According to Kinsey, the occurrence of bisexuals in society is not uncommon. Most grow up to have a normal heterosexual marriage and firmly suppress their homosexual tendency. The bisexual who is dissatisfied with a homosexual relationship and who wishes to fit into our culture's pattern of family and child rearing can frequently switch back to heterosexual relationships and have a successful marriage. But usually this reversal depends upon frank communication of his repressed homosexual fantasies so that he can control them in much the same way that a happily married heterosexual man may control his urge to have a secret affair with a reigning female sex symbol.

There is a variety of viewpoints and a great deal of controversy surrounding this issue. Discussions that should be scientific unfortunately often become political and moral. Anyone could be offended by a clinical attempt to understand the origin of their sexual preference, homosexual or heterosexual. Parents may certainly be offended by the notion that the way they reared their infant boy in the earliest months of his life is responsible for his sexual confusion. No matter what point of view is taken in this controversial area, there is bound to be debate and anger. Even among scientists, there are some who argue that it is all innate, and that environment has nothing to do with it. This point of view is frequently supported by the uncanny, repeatable phenomenon that homosexuals can trace their homosexual preference as far back into childhood as they can possibly remember. Homosexuals can literally never remember being anything but homosexual. But the clear-cut evidence from studies of intersex cases and transsexuals shows it to be much more probable that homosexual preference is a phenomenon intimately associated with early gender identity formation and sexual imprinting.

Just as transsexuals are usually not effeminate but rather truly feminine, most homosexuals are not openly effeminate. Furthermore, many men with mildly feminine mannerisms are not homosexual. There are many gradations and variations in gender confusion, and the mildest versions of these variations express themselves in all degrees of partial or complete homosexuality. Humans develop their sexual identity and sexual preference early in life, and the erotic imagery that is engraved in the brain during the first two years of life cannot be changed. The "macho" father who is afraid to show his infant son love and attention, thinking that only women should do that, or the father who just doesn't care at all, is far more likely to cause his son to grow up to be a homosexual than the father who lavishes affection upon his son. But awareness of homosexuality and open discussion of it at any stage of life will not in any way predispose anyone toward it.

Index

Illustrations are indicated by italics.

abdomen, testicles in. *See* testicles, undescended
adrenal gland, male hormone production in women by, 20, 21
adrenogenital syndrome, 178–79
age
  and differential diagnosis of torsion and epididymitis of testicle, 95–96
  of height of sexual responsiveness, 67
  See also aging
aging
  bed-wetting and, 127
  cancer of prostate and, 107–8
  enlargement of prostate and, *ix–x, xii,* 101–3
  erectile capability and, 15–16
  female sexuality and, 69–71
  male sexuality and, *xi,* 11–13, 16–17, 66–69
  testosterone levels and, 22–23
alarm wake-up device, bed-wetting and, 135, 138

alcoholics, male hormone production in, 36
5-Alpha reductase deficiency. *See* "penis at twelve" syndrome
ambiguous genitalia, 149–51, 165
  in adrenogenital syndrome, 179–80
  in otherwise normal boys, 157–58
  sex identity problems and, 156–57
  See also hermaphrodites; intersex children
animals
  bone in penises of, 8, 86
  sex drive in, 20–21
  sex reversals in, 197–98
  sexual seasonality in, 38–44
  testosterone injections in, 167–70
antibiotics
  in nonspecific urethritis, 63–64
  in syphilis, 60, 61
  See also tetracycline
athletes, testosterone and, 35–36
aversion therapy, sex offenders and, 30